Theory fo
Midwifery Practice

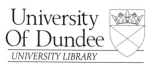

University
Of Dundee
UNIVERSITY LIBRARY

School of Nursing and Midwifery
Fife Campus

Date of Return

Theory for Midwifery Practice

ROSAMUND M. BRYAR

Department of Nursing and Midwifery
University of Wales Swansea

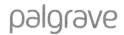

Published by
PALGRAVE
Houndmills, Basingstoke, Hampshire RG21 6XS and
175 Fifth Avenue, New York, N. Y. 10010
Companies and representatives throughout the world

PALGRAVE is the new global academic imprint of
St. Martin's Press LLC Scholarly and Reference Division and
Palgrave Publishers Ltd (formerly Macmillan Press Ltd).

ISBN 0–333–58867–3

This book is printed on paper suitable for recycling and made from fully managed and sustained forest sources.

A catalogue record for this book is available from the British Library.

10   9   8   7   6   5   4
07   06   05   04   03   02   01

Printed in Malaysia

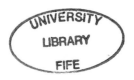

For my parents, Bernard Laurence
and Mary Forbes Bryar

CONTENTS

LIST OF TABLES

For me the writing of this book has been a journey, and I feel that I have come part of the way on that journey. My journey has been affected by my own questions, by the questions of others, by all the things that I have read and my knowledge and awareness of midwifery. Throughout this book the need for all midwives to clarify and try to state their beliefs and pictures of midwifery care is emphasised. Here I want to try to explain some of the questions I have had during the preparation of this book and some of the influences on my beliefs and picture of midwifery practice. My questions and concerns may be the same as yours, as you use this book in your own journey of thinking about midwifery practice, or your questions may be very different.

On the face of it I was not the ideal person to write a book such as this, about the development and use of theory or models in midwifery. I have never taught courses about the use of theory nor been greatly involved in the utilisation of models in midwifery or nursing practice except as a research midwife in the early 1980s at Queen Charlotte's Maternity Hospital. As a lecturer and external examiner I have been involved in the assessment of work using nursing models, both work in midwifery and different areas of nursing, but I have been largely an observer rather than a participant in the discussions about the use of models in midwifery or nursing. However, since my experience in the early 1980s, I had thought that there was a need for a book which considered theory development in midwifery but I had made no attempts to write such a book because of the reasons just given and because I realised the work that would be involved! In addition, my career had taken me away from midwifery back to primary health care.

When, unexpectedly, I was presented with the opportunity to prepare this book I realised that it was time someone had a go at it and, after some persuasion, I agreed. My aim has been to examine the basis of concept identification and theory development, to present information about work which has been done in this area in midwifery and to raise questions about this process. I was one of the early graduates from the Department of Nursing in Manchester, where Dr Dorothy Baker, Dr Charlotte Kratz, Emeritus Professor Baroness Jean McFarlane and Miss Norah Marsh ensured that we had the ability to go back to first principles and ask questions, and this is what I have tried to do in this book.

My first introduction to the use of theory in practice came early in my degree in Manchester in 1971 when Miss Marsh discussed with us Virginia Henderson's definition of nursing. This definition had a significant impact on me but I have little recollection of any other discussions of nursing theory in my degree, although we were encouraged to use the nursing process tool in recording our care. After I graduated I worked briefly in medical nursing, qualified as a midwife and worked as a health visitor. In none of these posts was there much discussion or evidence of the use of nursing/midwifery/health visiting theory in practice. It wasn't until I went to Queen Charlotte's Maternity Hospital as a research midwife in 1979 that I found myself thinking to any extent about the use of theory in practice.

The aim of the project at the hospital was to develop individualised care for childbearing women who were receiving care from the hospital. Much of the activity of the project was concentrated on changing parts of the organisation of the midwifery service to achieve continuity of care. For example, each woman was allocated to a midwife in the antenatal clinic who was then meant to see them on all subsequent clinic visits, and staff allocation rather than task allocation was introduced on the wards. In addition, care planning was introduced and this led us to consider models of care which could be utilised to underpin care planning. Due to the apparent lack of midwifery models, this consideration was of nursing models and the application of such models to midwifery. At that time little work had been done on the application of nursing models to midwifery and few midwives were familiar with nursing models. Given the extent of other changes that the project was seeking to introduce it was decided that a more pragmatic approach should be taken rather than trying to teach everyone about nursing models. In the event we held meetings with the midwives at which we tried to draw from them their model(s) of care. This process resulted in the midwifery assessment which can be seen as a very early, rather halting, attempt to crystallise some of the concepts underpinning midwifery practice. The project did not try to apply one model to midwifery care and midwives using the assessment and care plans largely applied their own personal, unstated models to the process of assessment and care planning.

Throughout this project there was a constant nagging problem. We never seemed able to discuss or question the actual care that was being given. The project was focused on changing organisational factors (but only those factors affecting midwifery practice) and introducing new recording systems but could not get near questions such as: What care was being given? What was the content of that care? What was the quality of that care? What was the thinking which lay behind that care? There was a general assumption that the care was good and that, once some organisational changes had been made, care would be individualised and continuity achieved.

Following the end of the project I worked for a while in Gloucester Maternity Hospital where I was given the much-needed opportunity to re-establish my clinical confidence. After this I became involved in education and returned to health visiting and primary health care research and development. It was in the field of research that my interest in the use of theory developed. In teaching research I became concerned with the lack of a theoretical base for much of the nursing and midwifery research I read and the lack of understanding among many nurses and midwives of the need for a theoretical framework for their research. Many people are still involved in constructing data-collection tools and collecting data without thinking about how that data relates to available knowledge and theory, the wider body of research and theory development which reduces the usefulness of their research. On the other hand, there is a growing body of qualitative research which does not start with a theoretical framework but aims to understand what is going on and develop theory from the data collected. There are, then, two traditions in research. The first uses available theory and knowledge to construct a theoretical framework which is investigated through research (deductive theorising) and the second starts with the (so-called) blank sheet – data is collected in relation to a phenomenon and theory is developed from that data (inductive theorising).

I therefore came to the task of thinking about theory in midwifery with a fairly open mind. I came to much of the literature on nursing models for the first time and found that in reading much of it I felt disquiet about four things. Firstly, my feelings of disquiet related to the lack of the presence of the individual nurse in the models. There was no reference to the personality of the nurse, the values, attitudes or needs of the nurse. My experience of midwifery and reading of midwifery literature made me feel that the personality of the midwife was vital and that there was a need in midwifery care for the midwife to understand her or himself. It was only when I re-read Carper (1992, originally published in 1978) that I began to find an answer to my disquiet in her discussion of personal knowledge and knowing the self. It was extremely reassuring to find that others were concerned with the person of the nurse. A paper by Taylor (1992) which discusses the need to re-identify nurses as human beings reinforced my feeling that awareness of the individual characteristics (the self) of the midwife should be discussed in a book on the use of models in midwifery.

My second feeling of disquiet about nursing models was the distance of many of the models from practice. Many of the most familiar nursing models are largely deductive theories which have been constructed from pre-existing models and theory, usually from disciplines outside nursing. These models present broad descriptions of ways of thinking about practice. They present broad descriptions of the relationship between concepts, and the research on testing the relationships between the concepts in the theories and models is patchy. These models and theories often seem to be very distant from everyday practice, and people seem to have to make a great deal of effort to apply these theories to practice. Reading Agyris and Schön (1974) helped me to see that what I was more concerned about were people's theories-in-use, the theories they use in their everyday practice or practice theory. It was this type of theory that had been troubling me during the project at Queen Charlotte's: how did the midwives actually undertake their practice? It was not sufficient to have descriptions of their theories-in-action, which espoused individualised care, when individualised care was self-evidently not being provided. Organisational theory and an understanding of the constraints on practice imposed by the organisation helped to explain the care provided, but this did not provide the full explanation. This could only be provided by an understanding of the theories-in-use which the midwives used to provide the care that was possible in that situation but which was not too dissonant with their own personal values about midwifery practice.

A third concern that I had about nursing models was the reaction that midwives would have to a book on the use of models in midwifery. One of my first thoughts about midwives and models was that midwives would have an antipathy to anything which was about the use of models. They would think that this is a book about the use of nursing models in midwifery, and to begin with, that is what I thought this book might be about. However, reading the literature showed me that there was a great deal more to the work of theory development in midwifery than the application of nursing models, important though that may be. One disappointment I have is that I have not been able to include some of the work that is currently progressing in Britain on theory development but which is as yet unpublished. I placed letters in a number of professional journals but these produced little response. Perhaps this publication will stimulate those who have undertaken work on theory development to publish their findings.

Finally, during the writing of this book I was fortunate to hear two eminent American nurse theorists talking at a conference, but what I heard filled me with fear, and it is this fear which is my last concern about the use of models in practice. Some nurse theorists seem to have gone so far down the path of existentialism that the everyday needs of the patient or childbearing woman seem to be lost in an understanding of the deeper self and needs of the individual, aspects of themselves which they themselves may not understand. The language used by some nurse theorists is extremely complicated and their meaning is often unclear. Language and the promotion of extreme philosophical positions creates a further barrier to our interest in thinking about how we practise. Much of the writing on models contributes to these barriers.

It has, however, been exciting to find that so much work has been undertaken on the development of theory in midwifery and nurse-midwifery practice contrary to much popular opinion on the subject. It has been particularly interesting to discover the work that has been done on theory testing, a vital part of the development of understanding of the relationship between midwifery actions and outcomes for the childbearing woman.

I hope that this book helps to reduce the barriers to thinking about theory and midwifery practice and helps you in your journey of understanding about how you think about midwifery and the care of the childbearing woman and her family. I have tried to explain how I have come this far on the journey. I now look forward to seeing how theory building in midwifery progresses in the future.

ROSAMUND BRYAR
Swansea

A whole host of people have helped in various ways with the writing of this book. My mother has borne the brunt of the effort and time that I have expended on this work and I thank her for her continued support, encouragement, patience and advice on use of the English language. Quentin, Siobhàn and Saoirse, my brother, his wife and young daughter have all provided me with much-needed support. Special thanks must go to Graham Evans of the University of Wales Swansea for advice and encouragement throughout the project. Four people whom I would also like to thank, Halle McCrae, Donna Mead, Ann Thomson and Edwin van Teijlingen, have given me particular help by reading and commenting on chapters. I would like to thank Halle McCrae for her encouragement. Donna Mead provided useful references, and discussion with her about Chapter 2 helped to clarify my thoughts. Ann Thomson provided, as usual, many challenging and helpful comments. Edwin van Teijlingen, in addition to his useful comments, has provided me with invaluable references and undertook the calculation in Chapter 3. A number of other people have provided particular help. I would like to thank Pam Hughes and Sandy Kirkman for early discussions; Joanna Brown typed some chapters and I would like to thank her for this and for her encouraging telephone calls; Chris Ruby for her encouragement and comments on one section; Hugh Price, Lecturer in Philosophy, for locating Socrates; Florence Telfer and Dorothy Carter for permission to use their unpublished work; Sally Pairman, Otago Polytechnic, New Zealand for permission to quote from the New Zealand handbook; Jon Meah and Chris Weeks, Babbage Designs, for the original art work on the diagrams and for their encouragement; Bill Bytheway for his general advice and Jo Alexander for getting me into this in the first place. I would like to thank my former colleagues at Teamcare Valleys (who could never quite understand my interest in midwifery) for their support and help in developing my thinking and my new colleagues in the midwifery teaching department of the Department of Nursing and Midwifery for their tolerance and helpful discussions about models. Many people have also contributed indirectly to the production of this book. These include the students on the Diploma in Midwifery in Cardiff, midwifery lecturers in the Mid Glamorgan College of Nursing and Midwifery and the Amman Valley Midwives, all of whom helped to keep me in contact with midwifery developments. The roots of this book lie in a project that was undertaken at Queen Charlotte's Maternity Hospital (1979–82) and I would like to thank all the midwives, students and other staff who were involved in that project and contributed so much to it. In particular I would like to thank Margaret Adams, Grace Strong and Mrs E. Ward who initiated the project. Kerry Lawrence, then Commissioning Editor at Macmillan, persuaded me to write this book – I hope it answers some of her questions about models and theory building. Finally, I would like to thank Barbara Green, Director of the Department of Nursing and Midwifery, University of Wales Swansea, for giving me the time to write.

A number of figures and tables have been reproduced in this book with the kind permission of the following:

Figure 2.2 with the permission of Macmillan Press Ltd.
Figure 3.1 with the permission of Heinemann Educational Books Ltd and Professor David Silverman.
Figure 6.3 with the permission of the American Journal of Nursing Company, 1988. *Reprinted from American Journal of Nursing*, Sept./Oct. 1988, Vol. 37, no. 5.
Figure 6.8 with the permission of Cambridge University Press.
Table 5.1 with the permission of Mark Allen Publishing Ltd.
Table 7.1 with the permission of Churchill Livingstone.

CHAPTER ONE

Introduction

Beyond this there is much that needs to be done in midwifery research and the subsequent development of midwifery concepts and theory. There is little time to do this, for the majority of midwives are now vastly limited in their practice by the nature of their setting. But midwifery researchers drawing upon the knowledge of those midwives who still retain a degree of autonomy in their practice could feed much of value into midwifery education, as well as raising our consciousness by showing us the nature of our own practice. (Kirkham, 1989, p. 136)

THEORY AND MIDWIFERY PRACTICE

The purpose of this first chapter is to set the scene for the discussion of theory development in midwifery, to identify the issues which will be considered and to outline the structure of the following chapters.

The word midwife means 'with woman'. We are all very familiar with this definition but what does it mean? Descriptions of midwives' activities with women identify midwives' empathy, their openness, their awareness of the feelings, thoughts and processes that women and their family are experiencing. Skills of observation are acute: the midwife watches patiently and with love; palpates and touches with sensitivity and kindness; listens with attention and time; smells with understanding and concern.

Midwives are described as special people with special attributes, wise women; in some cultures, only women who are mothers them-selves can become midwives. Even in Britain, many people who were already qualified nurses will remember the shock of being asked to find a responsible person to confirm that they were of good character before they could start learning to be a midwife. No one was that concerned about your character when you started your nursing course and no one said to you that to nurse was to be 'with patient'. No one suggested that your own self was of great significance as a nurse. Rather your own self was seen as more of a handicap. When you became 'too involved' with patients it was a cause for managerial concern and efforts had to be made to bring your character into line.

To be a midwife is to use the self, the person who is the midwife, in the practice of midwifery and the care of women and their families. Being a midwife becomes an inextricable part of the person who is called Mary, Gloria or Paul. The type of midwife that Mary, Gloria or Paul is, will depend on their personalities, experiences and beliefs but all, if they are 'good' midwives, will have as part of their natures the empathetic, intuitive, 'with woman' approach to midwifery practice. Midwifery identifies clearly that the practice of midwifery is dependent on the use of the self by the midwife. This identification of the self has always been of central importance in midwifery and is one of the ways that midwifery differs from nursing which has, until recently, been concerned with conformity and suppression of the individual.

Descriptions of midwifery practice and discussions with midwives emphasise the intuitive, the empathetic nature of the midwife's care and frequent comments are made about the lack of theory in midwifery, the lack of any models in midwifery and the fact that nursing models are not applicable to midwifery care. But here there seems to be a conflict with reality. The sensitive midwife who listens and hears, palpates and understands, observes and comprehends, uses her personal attributes but is able to collect and interpret information through the use of skills acquired through midwifery education and practice, to compare the information collected with knowledge and experience acquired through life, midwifery education and practice. Midwives have been provided with a surfeit of midwifery textbooks containing both experiential and research-based knowledge which describe the knowledge base of midwifery practice. Both Ina May Gaskin (1977) and Elizabeth Davis (1987), two empathetic and experiential midwives, emphasise the knowledge required to support women during childbearing in their respective books which can be categorised as textbooks of midwifery practice.

Textbooks describe, for example, physiological theories of labour and the production of breast milk; psychological theories of attachment and loss; sociological theories of social roles, and many others. If the day-to-day practice of Mary, Gloria or Paul is observed, they can be seen explaining the process of fetal development to parents, based on their knowledge of intrauterine growth; helping a woman decide on the appropriate method of pain relief, based on their knowledge of the physiology of labour and helping a father at home with his two year-old, based on their knowledge of theories of child development.

The ability of the midwife to 'be with' the woman and her family may be based on personal, empathetic, intuitive qualities, but the ability to help is based on the use of these qualities in combination with knowledge, with theory and with thinking about practice. In fact, this is the great achievement of the skilled, intuitive midwife: to be able to use the extensive knowledge base of midwifery and at the same time to care for the woman, her family and community in a sensitive, loving way. These midwives are the skilled, knowledge craftspeople who care for and love the tools and the medium with which they work.

Knowledge and theory at first appear to be anti-empathetic, anti-intuitive, anti-, in Elizabeth Davis's (1987) term, being open. Anti- all those attributes that midwives see as being central to midwifery care and anti- all the personal attributes that midwives feel they demonstrate in their care; that is, anti- our image of ourselves as people. This attitude says that you can either be empathetic, intuitive and 'with woman' or you can be a theorist, use models and thus be distant, detached from women. In fact those midwives who are intuitive, empathetic and who love and care for women are probably those who are most concerned to gain new knowledge, to read, to question, to undertake research. They are the midwives who, for example, have observed the effects of starvation in labour and have read research findings which demonstrate the need for adequate nutrition and will then make every effort to change hospital policies, often against great opposition. They have such concern for the women and families with whom they are involved that they feel the care they give must be based on the most up-to-date knowledge. This may be the most recent midwifery research about information needs in labour, physiological research about fetal blood circulation or it may be knowledge about complementary therapies which may relieve depression and stress in pregnancy. Whatever the discipline or source of knowledge, these midwives are concerned to provide the most effective care for women.

These midwives are also concerned to develop knowledge. Through their empathetic observation of women throughout the childbearing process they build up a huge stock of knowledge about the process of childbearing and needs of women and through this process develop practice theory. Through a process of reflection, further observation and more reflection, they are able to make predictions about the type of care which will be most suitable for which women under what circumstances and can put forward theories of practice. They are able, in research and theory-building terms, to make statements about causal relationships between concepts. They can make statements, for example, about the relationship between immersion in water in the first stage of labour and dilatation of the cervix and pain relief. Their close observation and concern makes it possible for them to make such statements which they, and others, can then test and develop into models or theories of midwifery care (see Chapter 2).

It seems to me that this is the essence of the art of midwifery: informed intuition, informed empathy. Empathy that is uninformed by theory, knowledge and reflective thinking is, at its best, sympathy and support that does no harm; at its worst, sympathy and failure to recognise serious problems that require skilled action. The midwife who is empathetic but lacks up-to-date knowledge, who does not think about and reflect on day-to-day practice, is unable to be fully 'with woman' and exercise the art of midwifery.

The denial of the use of theory is the first paradox in midwifery with which this book will be concerned. The other paradox central to this book is the conflict between the rhetoric of midwifery and the reality of practice in many settings in Britain and many other industrialised countries today. As described earlier, the rhetoric of midwifery identifies the closeness of the relationship between women and midwives, but the reality is often very different. In reality, the majority of midwives work within organisations that are based on a medical model of care and may themselves hold a medical-model approach to care. Research and anecdotal evidence indicates that women feel that their needs are not met by care provided within this model (Oakley, 1979; 1980). There are many reasons why midwives adopt a medical-model approach to care, which will be explored later, but the education of midwives and the settings within which most work are two factors of central importance.

Kitzinger (1988), rather controversially, uses the term 'nurse-midwives' to describe all those midwives who were qualified as nurses before they commenced their education as midwives and it should be remembered that this applies to the majority of midwives in Britain today. Preparation as nurses within educational systems which have been based in the bio-physical medical model has had a significant effect on the ways of thinking adopted by midwives. This has been transferred to their practice as midwives, although some midwives would argue that socialisation in midwifery has counteracted attitudes developed during socialisation as a nurse.

The organisational setting is of great significance in affecting the type of care that is provided and the way that midwives practice. Benoit (1987; 1989) provides very clear evidence of this in her study of the different settings in which midwives practice or practised in the past in Newfoundland and Labrador. Currently in Britain, efforts are being made to change the organisation of midwifery care to enable women to experience continuity, choice and control (Department of Health, 1993a and 1993b). As these changes take place it is necessary for midwives to examine their own models of practice and to consider to what extent the new organisations, such as teams or midwifery-led units, are based on a midwifery model. Such consideration should include an evaluation and understanding of the medical model and the effects of perpetuation of this model within new organisations. New organisations, as old organisations, reflect the models of care held by those working within them so that those working in new organisations need to make their models, or pictures of care, very clear to themselves, to women and everyone with whom they are working. Hughes (1988) asks: 'How can "models" challenge the constraints which thwart good midwifery now?' (p. 2). It is the contention, and the challenge of this book, that it is by making personal and shared midwifery values explicit that midwives can talk and think about the essence of midwifery care and contribute to the building of organisations which will meet the wider needs of women. Without this discussion and debate there is a danger that the care experienced by women will continue to be based unconsciously on models of care which do not meet the full range of social, psychological, developmental, educational and physical needs of women. Without this discussion, midwives working within new organisations, as well as those continuing to work in more traditional settings, may continue to feel frustrated that their personal models still conflict with the organisational model and may feel that no real change has taken place. Consideration of the values and models held by individuals and the constraints of the organisation on those models may help to identify places within the organisation where pressure for change may be applied to achieve real change in the care provided.

Skilled midwifery care results from the combination of the personal qualities of the midwife with knowledge, theory, reflection and thinking about how theory and knowledge can be best used in the care of the individual woman. Theory provides the tools for the job. Theory provides a structure within which midwives can compare the present experiences of the woman they are caring for with the responses identified in the theory. Theory for practice sensitises midwives to the things that they should be watching for and helps to identify those factors which are central from those factors that are less important. The use of theory involves the comparison of the experiences of the woman with knowledge and theory from midwifery practice and from a range of disciplines. Midwives make this comparison through thinking about women and thinking about the theories they hold about the behaviour and needs of women. This thinking leads to the development of practice theory and theories for practice. The quality of the thinking that midwives undertake will have a direct effect on their actions, their care of the woman, her family and the community.

Schön (1992) argues for artistry in practice and the titles of midwifery textbooks refer to the art as well as the science of midwifery practice (Silverton, 1993). But there is little description or definition of this art; the implication is that midwives somehow 'have it'. It is true that there are many midwives who display intuition and empathy, who know the right things to say, who seem to know, before a woman or her partner asks, what is needed at a particular moment. In other fields there are artists, writers and craftspeople who have exceptional talents and create unique, beautiful paintings, books or furniture. Some of these people are self-taught, having learnt to paint, for example, through a process of trial and error, while others have spent many years studying the processes involved in painting, understanding colour, perspective, technique. These artists combine this knowledge with their talent to produce unique works of art. The knowledge they are using may not be explicit to them as they paint, as it has become a part of the way they paint, but at times it may become explicit. For example, when an artist is trying to create a particular colour, different pigments may be combined based on the artist's knowledge and recall of that knowledge. The knowledge enables the artist to reproduce the same colour over and over again in circumstances where that colour is required (a theory of practice). In the same way the artist creates knowledge or a theory of which combinations of pigments will produce what colours. This is done through the practice of making colours, through the practice of painting (a practice theory). This personal theory then becomes part of the knowledge base of the painter from which the painter can draw in the creation of future paintings. This type of theory is described by Agyris and Schön (1974) as theory-in-use and by observing the practice of the painter, or the midwife, we can identify their theories-in-use.

As with the artist, much midwifery practice is based on the intuitive, personal talent of the individual midwife, but care can only be enhanced if midwives are able to articulate their theories and knowledge base. This articulation enables the utilisation of strategies of care which will best meet the particular needs of the individual woman and helps to ensure that needs are not overlooked. As with the artist who is able to predict the colour that will be produced, the clearer articulation of the theory underpinning midwifery care may help to clarify the outcomes of midwifery care: 'there is some information on the structures of associated services but very little is known about the content of care and just exactly what does or does not affect pregnancy outcomes' (World Health Organization, 1985a, p. 1).

This book is about this process of thinking about care. Midwifery care is essentially practical and much of the learning about midwifery focuses on the development of practical, interpersonal skills. These skills are developed through a process which must include thinking. But less attention has been paid to the process of thinking and the need for reflection and the development of midwifery theory than to the actual doing of midwifery. This is an experience not unique to mid-wifery. In many scientific disciplines in past centuries, developments were largely based on thinking about phenomena but today much scientific work is completely involved with experimentation and the collection of data. There has been an explosion in the collection of data and a neglect of reflection and thinking about the types of data to collect and thinking about that data once collected.

Socrates, the son of a midwife, in Plato's *Theaetetus* (Cornford, 1946) describes himself as a midwife of ideas, helping others to bring forth ideas, but not himself giving birth to ideas, in the same way that a midwife helps a woman to give birth:

My art of midwifery is in general like theirs; the only difference is that my patients are men, not women, and my concerns are not with the body but with the soul that is in travail of birth. And the highest point of my art is the power to prove by every test whether the off-spring of a young man's thought is a false phantom or instinct with life and truth. I am so far like the midwife, that I cannot myself give birth to wisdom; and the common reproach is true, that, though I question others, I can myself bring nothing to light because there is no wisdom in me. The reason is this: heaven constrains me to serve as a midwife, but has debarred me from giving birth. So of myself I have no sort of wisdom, nor has any discovery ever been born to me as the child of my soul. (Cornford, 1946, p. 26)

The aim of this book is to help midwives, women as well as men, if not to become philosophers, to ask questions, to think about their practice, about the theory that informs their practice and the theory that may arise from their practice. Hughes (1988) has called for a debate on the place of theory in midwifery practice, and this book hopes to contribute to that debate through raising questions and topics for discussion.

Midwives need to clarify 'where they are coming from', to make explicit to themselves and to others the basis for their practice: the values, attitudes, skills and knowledge that combine in midwifery care. This book is an aid to this process. It aims to help midwives think about the basis of their practice and the conditions that are necessary for midwifery care; to help in the thinking about the underlying concepts or theories of practice and to consider the use of those concepts or theories in the tools they use in their everyday practice. Much of this underlying theory and the concepts of everyday practice are generally hidden from discussion and from view, sometimes even hidden from the person who holds them! If these theories, concepts and models can be identified and discussed, they form a way of aiding communication between midwives, the childbearing woman and her family, and other practitioners, helping to identify shared meanings and values.

One way of clarifying the meaning of midwifery care is to examine the basis and context of care:

- How do I think about women and about myself as a woman (or a man)?
- What are the needs of women in the process of childbearing, childbirth and later in child rearing?
- Do I consider all the needs that women and their families may have or do I tend to focus on one area of need?
- If I focus on one area, why is that?
- What knowledge do I use in caring for women?
- What constraints do I experience from day to day in caring for childbearing women?
- What is the contribution of other members of the multidisciplinary team to the care of the childbearing woman and her child?
- How much responsibility do I want?
- How much responsibility do women want?
- How do I help women exercise control in their care?
- What are my views about care; empowerment; choice; holism; equality and continuity?
- What are the views of my midwifery and other colleagues about these concepts? Do we share the same views? Have we ever discussed them?

In this book the aim is to discuss these and other questions, to work towards an understanding of the context of midwifery care, to consider the need for shared meanings or, at least, the discussion of different meanings and ways of putting these shared meanings into practice through the utilisation of models and theories of caring and practice.

You will by now have identified another aim of this book – which is that it aims to be interactive! It is essential for a book about thinking that the reader thinks! I cannot know the values that you hold: you have to bring them to the surface yourself. I cannot reflect on your practice for you: you have to do that. I cannot know the context within which you practice midwifery: you have to identify the supports and constraints there yourself. I cannot know the theories that you have developed from your own practice: you have to describe them yourself. All I can do is bring together material which I hope will help you in your thinking about midwifery practice (or action) and the theory underpinning that practice. This material will help you to consider the theoretical tools that you use in your practice and may contribute to making these theories more coherent to yourself and to others. Your thinking about these issues will then contribute to the wider debate within midwifery and the search for a language or languages for midwifery practice.

The central contention of this book is that thinking affects practice: that the mental pictures that we each hold affect our practice and that the mental pictures underpinning the organisations within which we work and provide care (and which we may or may not share) have a profound effect on the care experienced by childbearing women. This book seeks to help clarify the question: How do I care? How do you care?

ORGANISATION OF THE BOOK

There are two themes which permeate this book: the role of the midwife and the needs of the childbearing woman. It is the premise of the book that a clearer understanding of the concepts, theories and models which inform midwifery care will result in a better understanding of the role of the midwife and the type of care that women need. All the chapters are therefore concerned with the process of clarifying and identifying these concepts, theories and models. Exercises at the end of each chapter may be undertaken by individuals or groups as part of the process of clarification.

A few points need to be made about the use of language. Midwives may be female or male and efforts have been made to refer to midwives in the plural to avoid identification of midwives as female or male. The identification of midwives as female has only occurred when discussing midwifery practice in periods or countries where it is or was an exclusively female activity.

Secondly, much of the work on concept identification and theory building in midwifery has taken place in the United States of America. Midwifery in that country has been severely restricted by medical practice and people who practice midwifery describe themselves as nurse-midwives. The inclusion of the term nurse in their description of themselves raises antipathy among midwives in Britain who, especially in more recent times, have sought to distance themselves from nursing.

Wiedenbach (1960) provides an explanation of the use of this term referring to the negative attributes associated with the term midwife in the USA where it was associated with the practice of: 'a well-intentioned, but uneducated, old woman' (p. 256). While many would argue with this interpretation of history, this prevailing attitude in society contributed to the adoption of the term nurse-midwife in the USA. More controversially still, Wiedenbach (1960) argues for the inclusion of the word nurse in the title as, she argues, midwifery may be considered synonymous with obstetrics: the midwife being the practitioner in normal obstetrics. On this basis the nurse-midwife in Wiedenbach's (1960) analysis straddles two professions: nursing and medicine, and this is reflected in the use of the title nurse-midwife in the USA. This viewpoint will not sit comfortably with British midwives; however, the different pressures and constraints under which nurse-midwives practise in the USA has to be acknowledged. In the following the term nurse-midwife is used when reference is being made to literature from the USA rather than substituting this term with midwife and midwifery.

Another controversy in midwifery lies around the use of the term patient to describe the childbearing woman. The use of this term implies adherence to a medical model of care and for this reason it is rejected by many. Throughout this book the term patient has been avoided except where quotations have been made from other sources in which the term patient is used. It is interesting when considering the literature reviewed in this book to recognise the extent to which the term patient is used by midwives and others writing about care of the childbearing woman. Use of this term can be said to demonstrate an aspect of the model of midwifery care held by those writers.

In Chapter 2 some of the terms, such as theory, philosophy, models and concepts, are explored and defined. The central concepts which inform the practice of midwifery are also considered along with the process of developing theory. The organisational context of midwifery care is considered in Chapter 3 and a model discussed, the action approach to organisations, which helps to relate together the different elements that affect care (the action). These elements are the attitudes and knowledge in the wider society; factors relating to the structures and role relationships within an organisation, and the knowledge and attitudes (the mental pictures) held by midwives and others within the organisation and by childbearing women and their families. This model is then used to underpin the discussions in the later chapters. This chapter also includes a discussion of the difficulties of achieving change and the need for individuals to have time to work through change. The organisation of maternity services in the Netherlands is described as an example of the influence an alternative model of childbearing may have on the organisation of maternity services.

Chapter 4 considers some models, a theory and a concept which inform the knowledge and attitudes in the wider society. Midwifery, as discussed above, is influenced by a whole range of disciplines and the different models, theories and concepts of those disciplines. To provide examples of this process, two models, a theory and a concept which influence the environment of midwifery care are explored: the medical model, the Health for All model, bonding theory and the concept of participation. Consideration of these models, theory and concept indicate the power of different models and the wide effects changes in the model or theory informing care has on that care. This consideration of underlying theory is particularly important at a time when maternity services are being focused on the provision of choice, continuity and control as central outcomes of care. There is a need to explore the models, theories and concepts that will make a reality of that care.

Chapters 5, 6 and 7 are concerned with the mental pictures (personal models and theories) that midwives have of their practice. Chapter 5 considers the evidence from midwifery literature of the philosophies, theories and models held by midwives. These philosophies can be seen to lie at different points on the continuum between the model of pregnancy as a normal life event and the medical model of pregnancy, and this chapter ends with a discussion of this continuum. In Chapter 6 the work of five theorists who have examined the care of childbearing women and devised theories to help understand and guide this care is presented. Four of these theorists are American nurse-midwives and it is interesting to speculate about the reasons for the extent of theory development in the USA, given the small numbers of nurse-midwives. Also included in this chapter is the work of a British midwife which is implicitly concerned with theory development.

Chapter 7 describes the work that has taken place in Britain on the application of models from nursing to midwifery and other activities which are contributing to the development of theory and model building in midwifery. The final chapter, Chapter 8, is concerned with the process of understanding and developing practice theory and theories of practice. This chapter discusses deductive and inductive approaches to theory and model building which may be used by midwives to develop understanding of the basis of midwifery care.

Summary

In this chapter some of the issues have been raised which need to be considered in any discussion of theory building. Some of the paradoxes in midwifery thinking have also been identified and it has been argued that midwifery theory needs to be thought about and placed centrally in any discussions of midwifery practice. The interactive nature of this book has been presented. Having reached the end of the book the reader who undertakes the activities should have a clearer idea of their own models and theories of and for midwifery practice. Finally the structure of the book was described.

Activities

Before going on to the next chapters consider the content of this introductory chapter and think about the following issues which will form a basis for your own exploration of your own personal models and theories of midwifery practice through the remainder of this book.

1 How do I think about women and about myself as a woman (or a man)?
2 What are the needs of women in the process of childbearing, childbirth and later in child rearing?
3 Do I consider all the needs that women and their families may have or do I tend to focus on one area of need? If I focus on one area, why is that?
4 What knowledge do I use in caring for women?
5 What constraints do I experience from day to day in caring for childbearing women?
6 What is the contribution of other members of the multidisciplinary team to the care of the childbearing woman and her child?
7 How much responsibility do I want?
8 How much responsibility do women want?
9 How do I help women exercise control in their care?
10 What are my views about care; empowerment; choice; holism; equality and continuity?
11 What are the views of my midwifery and other colleagues about these concepts? Do we share the same views? Have we ever discussed them?

CHAPTER TWO

Thinking about midwifery

But how do you teach something so personal? Are you trying to foster a new Isadora? 'You can't teach anyone to be the way Isadora was. Nobody could do that. But there's a technique and there's the dances that have been passed down.' This determined talk of technique gives the lie to the popular belief that Isadora Duncan made it up as she went along. This was never the case; she spent weeks rehearsing in draughty studios with her indefatigable mother at the upright. So why do people imagine it was unrehearsed? Because it looked so easy when she did it – I imagine – and because she was so spontaneous people thought it was improvised. But Isadora had a sense of humour: people had already started saying: 'There's no technique in it', so with her sense of humour she probably encouraged people to think that. (Levene, 1993, p. 10)

INTRODUCTION

The purpose of this chapter is to consider some of the words and ideas used in thinking about practice. What is meant by the terms: philosophy, paradigm, conceptual model, theory, concept? How do these terms relate to each other? Where does theory come from and how is it described? How can an understanding of these terms contribute to the understanding of day-to-day practice of the midwife and how can this enhance the experience a woman has of midwifery care?

On the face of it, the idea that this chapter should provide a description of the above terms appears unproblematic and commendable. However, the task is made more difficult by the vast range of literature on nursing models and theory development, the growing literature on theory development in midwifery and the confusion in this literature of the different terms. Taking one example, Carveth (1987) appears to use two different definitions of conceptual model within one article on building conceptual models for nurse-midwifery. On the one hand she refers to the personal model of practice held by the individual midwife as a 'conceptual model' while also referring to extremely abstract representations which: 'cannot be tested, or observed' (Carveth, 1987, p. 22) as conceptual models. Robinson (1992) has described the pain and effort involved in the mental process of concept development and this same effort has been required in the process of determining the meaning of different terms used by different authors when discussing theory development.

The following discussion is based on an interpretation of some of the literature on this subject and the reader is referred to the texts for more detailed descriptions of the ways in which the various authors describe these terms. Many texts are devoted to discussion of the meaning and understanding of conceptual models and theory building in nursing. British texts include Chapman (1985), Aggleton and Chalmers (1986; 1987), Kershaw and Salvage (1986), Webb (1986), Pearson and Vaughan (1986) and Kitson (1993). American texts include Fawcett (1984), Marriner-Tomey (1989), Fitzpatrick and Whall (1989), Moody (1990) and Chinn and Kramer (1991). Classic American articles on the development of theory in nursing since the early 1960s have been brought together in one volume (Nicholl, 1992). Articles on the development of theory in midwifery include those by Hughes (1988), Bryar (1988), Smith (1991), Spires (1991) and Price and Price (1993). American articles and books on the development of theory in nurse-midwifery include those by Mercer (1986), Carveth (1987), Thompson *et al.* (1989) and Fawcett *et al.* (1993). Some of this literature is referred to in the following discussion while the work of some of the midwifery and nurse-midwifery theorists is discussed in more depth in later chapters (see Chapters 6 and 7).

THINKING UNDERPINNING PRACTICE

When a midwife undertakes any activity or action, provides care, be it psychological, educational or physical, that activity is undertaken in the light of the midwife's personal understanding, knowledge and theories. Firstly, the midwife has to have an understanding of the need or problem which requires attention. This understanding will be based on previous experience of such needs and what has been previously learnt about such needs (the knowledge base). The midwife will be able to state or define the need. Next, the midwife will have an understanding of the action which might alleviate the problem or reduce the need. Midwives will also have an understanding of their ability or the ability of their colleagues to meet the need.

For example, if a woman is experiencing a primary post-partum haemorrhage it is known that she will have a range of physiological needs relating to sudden blood-loss. She will also have psychological needs relating to anxiety about her own safety, concerns for her newborn baby and partner. It is known that immediate action has to be taken to halt the haemorrhage and restore fluid balance. Midwives will also know that they will need the assistance of obstetric colleagues to care for the woman in this emergency situation. At the same time the woman and her partner must be provided with support and information.

The actions carried out in this situation, the efforts to halt the haemorrhage, are preceded by thought which brings together the knowledge needed to meet and respond to the situation. If one of the elements is omitted in the actions, the care provided may be less satisfactory. For example, if the haemorrhage is stopped but no attempt made to restore fluid balance the woman may suffer further complications. Or if treatment is provided without adequate reassurance to the woman or her partner, one or both may suffer long-term anxieties about the possibility of haemorrhage at subsequent births.

This thinking about the action provides a theory about the best way of meeting the need (practice theory). Thinking about the outcome of the actions, how quickly the woman recovered, the way that different members of the health team worked together or the woman's reaction to her care can lead to modification and development of the theory which can then be tested and developed further in other practical situations where haemorrhage occurs. In this way a practice theory becomes a theory of or for practice. The thinking and reflection on this recent incident, combined with information from earlier incidents, may help to overcome one problem about this approach to theory development, which is the influence of more recent events or experiences on practice. More recent events will be more clear in the memory and the theory developed following these events may be applied to the present experience of haemorrhage. However, it may be that the present haemorrhage may be more similar to other haemorrhages experienced some time ago and the theory developed following these experiences may be more appropriate to the present care. In-depth reflection, which brings together theory from past experiences with theory developed from the present experience, will integrate the knowledge from this range of experiences and ameliorate the effect of recency.

In this example the midwife has brought together pre-existing knowledge combined with previous experience to provide a theory of what action should be taken to enable immediate, appropriate care to be provided. Agyris and Schön (1974) describe this type of theory as a theory-in-use and it is this type of theory (practice theory) which Benner and Wrubel (1989) seek to expose in descriptions of exemplars of nursing practice. Luker (1988) describes these models as working models which the individual nurse or midwife uses in their own practice. Theory, in this sense, is intimately bound up with practice being developed from the articulation of the practice of midwifery or nursing and is termed practice theory (Pearson, 1992). This description demonstrates the use of two types of theory in practice: the use of knowledge from other disciplines and knowledge derived from practice, practice theory or theory-in-use. This description excludes reference to another type of the theory, derived from the general or grand models of nursing, which may be the type of theory which comes to mind when theory development in midwifery is discussed.

Chinn and Kramer (1991) comment that in recent years there has been a shift in nursing theory towards the development of practice and research-based theory, away from the more general or grand 'theories' (conceptual models) of nursing. This differentiation of two forms of theory development is important for an understanding of the development and role of theory in midwifery. Chinn and Kramer (1991) provide a summary of the development of nursing theory from 1952 to 1981 which includes descriptions of the general or grand 'theories' (conceptual models) of nursing developed by theorists including Roy, Orem, Wiedenbach, Neuman and many others.

Reference is frequently made to the lack of general or grand-model development in midwifery. While examination of the work of a number of theorists in later chapters will show that this view is not necessarily supported, it is still the case that there is little evidence of the development of grand theories in midwifery. In contrast, midwives and nurse-midwives appear to have concentrated on understanding practice and midwives have called for theory that is based in practice (Kirkham 1989; Price and Price, 1993). There is also evidence that some nurse-midwives have begun to develop and test middle-range predictive theories of midwifery practice (Lehrman, 1989).

It is interesting to speculate why midwives may have taken this approach to theory development in contrast to their nursing colleagues. Price and Price (1993) suggest that theory development has occurred in nursing for a number of reasons which relate to professional development and boundary maintenance, graduate education and defence of nursing practice in the face of more recent financial pressures on the employment of skilled, highly-qualified nurses. It may be argued that the professional position of midwives has been under pressure for so long that midwives may not have seen theory development as a means of professional development until the recent renaissance in midwifery (House of Commons Health Committee, 1992). It may also be suggested that midwives may have always been more concerned with the practice of midwifery rather than theorising about that care. The grand or general models of nursing, because of their very generality, may appear to lack immediate practical relevance and this may also have deterred midwives from developing models for midwifery along similar lines. Midwives, in this sense, may then be seen to have leapfrogged the grand-model development stage that nurses have been involved with during the last 30 years and to have moved to the stage of developing or, in Smith's (1991) term, discovering practice theory which is now the growing focus also of nursing theory development (Benner and Wrubel, 1989). Some of the terms used in this process of thinking about, or theorising about, practice will now be discussed.

PHILOSOPHY

Philosophy is a discipline which is concerned with exploring and postulating explanations for reality (Chinn and Kramer, 1991). There are a large number of philosophical approaches to this thinking about reality, including religious traditions, Marxism, existentialism and phenomenology (Pearson and Vaughan, 1986; Rhodes, 1988), but in relation to thinking about midwifery practice the need is for each midwife to identify their personal philosophy or philosophies of life and midwifery practice. These philosophies will, of course, be based on wider philosophies or ways of describing reality found in the general community as the midwife is a person, as well as a midwife, and the attitudes, values and beliefs that midwives hold result from their membership of a particular community and society as well as from their secondary socialisation into the world of midwifery practice. Pearson and Vaughan (1986) describe a philosophy as both the pursuit of knowledge and a description of personal beliefs:

> So philosophy can be interpreted as the pursuit of wisdom or knowledge about the things around us and what causes them. A philosophy is an explicit statement about what you believe and about what values you hold. These values and beliefs will, in turn, affect the way you behave. (Pearson and Vaughan, 1986, p. 8)

In recent years there has been a great deal of activity in midwifery units and teams to generate ward, unit or team 'philosophies' and some of these are discussed in Chapter 5. Downe (1991) has commented on this in relation to the process of standard-setting and urges midwives to avoid the simplistic notion of devising a 'philosophy for midwifery' which is forgotten once it is filed in the procedure book but to think honestly about their beliefs and values, their philosophy, and the consequences of their philosophy for care:

> It [the midwife's philosophy] must be an expression of our honest thoughts about what midwifery means to us. For example, if we use a medical model, what are the consequences for the women we serve? Are they different if we use a midwifery model of care? (Downe, 1991, p. 3)

Downe (1991) emphasises the need to make beliefs about midwifery practice explicit. One way to do this is to consider the types of knowledge that combine to make up the philosophy that the midwife might hold of midwifery care. Carper (1992) (in an article originally published in 1978) describes four types of knowledge which underpin the practice of nursing: empirics, nursing science; aesthetics, the art of nursing; personal knowledge; and ethics, the moral component.

Nursing science is described as the knowledge and theories about nursing which explain and inform nursing care. This knowledge is in the process of being developed, so that it is not possible to say that nursing shares one common world-view or paradigm to explain nursing practice. Carper (1992) uses the example of the change in the definition of health, to a definition which sees health as more than the absence of disease, as an example of a radical rethinking of health, which is now thought of as a process or continuum rather than a static state. This way of thinking about health then leads to new possibilities for interventions by the nurse (or midwife) to support people to move along the health continuum.

The aesthetic component in nursing is more difficult to describe and, Carper suggests, has been given less attention in nursing as this type of knowing is associated with the (now-deprecated) apprenticeship system of learning in which (under the best circumstances) the student gained knowledge about the less tangible aspects of care from observation and interaction with skilled practitioners. As suggested in Chapter 1, this type of knowing, the art of midwifery, is expressed in the intuitive actions of the midwife but may be difficult to express verbally. This type of knowing is shown in the process of empathy or in the role-taking with patients or the childbearing woman which is a component of Riehl's Interactionist Model of Nursing (see Chapter 7) (Aggleton and Chalmers, 1986).

Rhodes (1988) (writing from the American perspective) argues strongly for the recognition of the aesthetic component of nurse-midwifery practice and for the study of the philosophy of aesthetics. She comments:

> Through aesthetics we can come to understand the various meanings of 'art' and begin to apply these concepts to scholarly and clinical work. It is the art of nurse-midwifery that will distinguish us from other obstetrical/gynecologic practitioners and philosophically make our research nurse-midwifery research. We must begin to explicate in scholarly works the value and relationship of aesthetics to the discipline of nurse-midwifery and nurse-midwifery practice. (Rhodes, 1988, p. 284)

While Rhodes (1988) comments that the notion of aesthetics may seem strange, many practitioners, and many childbearing women, will be able to describe the art they have experienced in their own care and in the care provided by others.

The third type of knowledge that Carper (1992) describes is personal knowledge. This type of knowledge is considered the most difficult to articulate but is concerned with the individual nurse's or midwife's knowledge of themselves: 'Personal knowledge is concerned with the knowing, encountering and actualizing of the concrete, individual self. One does not know about the self; one strives simply to know the self' (Carper, 1992, p. 220). Carper (1992) considers that this personal knowledge is vital if nurses are going to be able to avoid objectifying patients and to use themselves in the therapeutic relationship. Midwives whose philosophy of themselves is that they should be open and should express themselves with women for whom they are caring will clearly provide different care from midwives whose view is that a more detached attitude should be taken (see Chapter 5).

Taylor (1992) argues that this type of knowledge, the nature of the nurse as a person or human being, has been largely ignored in the development of nursing models and theory. This author suggests that much of the literature on nursing and patients describes patients and nurses as having different characteristics and fails to acknowledge the human qualities that patients and nurses share. Nurses are seen as bringing special knowledge and skills to patient care but their shared experiences as human beings are ignored. She comments: 'Do nurses and patients relate only in terms of needs and goals? Is that all they are?' (Taylor, 1992, p. 1046) and suggests: 'that it is possible for nurses not only to be knowledgeable and skillful but to be all the more therapeutic when they are in touch with, and live out, their own ordinariness in their day-to-day working lives' (Taylor, 1992, p. 1046).

This dehumanisation of the nurse may be contrasted with the position in midwifery where, possibly because of the emotion surrounding the process of birth, it seems less possible for the self of the midwife to be ignored. This type of knowledge, personal knowledge, it may be suggested, is a key part of the philosophy of the midwife. The lack of attention to this type of knowledge in nursing conceptual models may be one reason why midwives have found such models lack relevance in their lives and their work, their care of the childbearing woman. This personal knowledge may then be a concept that is an essential element of a model of midwifery.

However, as discussed in Chapter 1, a paradox is evident in midwifery between the close relationship that is advocated between the midwife and the woman and the reality of care experienced by many women and the reality of practice for many midwives who have not been able to 'get close' to women either because of organisational constraints or attitudes developed during their occupational education. Nursing and midwifery practice is fraught with anxiety (which in the case of midwifery practice is reinforced by the obstetric/medical model of pregnancy). Menzies (1970) has discussed the means that nurses working in the hospital organisation use to control this anxiety. Methods used include splitting of the nurse–patient relationship, through task allocation and splitting of care between many departments; depersonalisation of the nurse and the patient, exemplified by reference to patients by their disease; detachment and denial of feelings; ritual task performance; the upward reference of responsibility to higher layers in the hierarchy and other means. These features are also present in the organisation of maternity services. In nursing, new methods of work organisation including primary nursing and a growing interest in the therapeutic aspects of the nurse–patient interaction have challenged these traditional defence mechanisms and the emotional labour involved in caring for patients and in working with other colleagues in health care settings has been described (Smith, 1992). Similarly, in midwifery the development of team midwifery and the emphasis on continuity of care suggests a need to examine traditional defence mechanisms and ways that may be needed to support midwives in their closer relationships with childbearing women, possibly through peer support or different means of supporting reflection on practice (Morton-Cooper and Palmer, 1993).

The final type of knowledge that Carper (1992) describes is ethical knowledge. This type of knowledge is concerned with moral codes and provides the basis for ethical decision-making in practice. Combined together these four types of knowing (midwifery science, the art of midwifery, the personal knowledge of the midwife and the ethical, moral component) describe and demonstrate the values, beliefs and philosophy of care held by the individual midwife.

Clarification of these four patterns of knowing may assist midwives in articulating their philosophies of midwifery care and of life. This is an essential first step in describing practice theories, which will be fundamentally affected by personal philosophies; in choosing between pre-existing conceptual models, some of which will be closer to one's own personal philosophy than others, and in developing models for midwifery care.

CONCEPTUAL MODELS

Conceptual models provide an abstract representation of the ideas upon which a discipline is based. Conceptual models or conceptual frameworks of nursing are: 'abstract models of what nursing is, or *should* be.' (Aggleton and Chalmers, 1986, p. 4). Conceptual models are constructed in various ways but may bring together information and insights from a variety of disciplines, from personal and general philosophies, from observation of practice and from research, to help provide a framework within which practice, education and research in a discipline can be better understood and around which these three activities can be organised.

Fawcett (1992) (in an article originally published in 1980) which aims to: 'provide a clear definition of conceptual models' (p. 424), defines a conceptual model as follows: 'The term conceptual model, and synonymous terms such as conceptual framework, system, or scheme, refer to global ideas about the individuals, groups, situations and events of interest to a science' (Fawcett, 1992, p. 425) and comments that: 'Conceptual models usually evolve from the intuitive insights of scientists, often initially within the frame of reference of a related discipline' (Fawcett, 1992, p. 426).

This process of model development is clearly shown in descriptions of the development of nursing models by nursing theorists, such as Henderson, Roy and Orem as well as in discussions of the writings of Florence Nightingale which are seen as the first work on model building in nursing (Fitzpatrick and Whall, 1989; Marriner-Tomey, 1989).

Models provide a framework for understanding and developing practice, for guiding actions, for organising education and identifying research questions to be asked. Conceptual models may be represented in various ways: as mental models, physical models or symbolic models (Lancaster and Lancaster, 1992). A mental model is described in language which identifies the relationships between concepts. A physical model may be a representation of reality, for example, an architect's model of a birth centre which demonstrates in physical terms the ways in which the model facilitates choice (alternative facilities), privacy, continuity and other important concepts. A symbolic model may be in the form of a diagram, mathematical formulation or other representation. The diagrams showing the onset and development of uterine contractions relating to the concepts of nerve functions, muscle fibres and hormonal influences are an example of such a conceptual model.

Robinson (1992) argues with the comparison that is sometimes made between nursing models and other models such as those described above and suggests that while nurses and midwives use such models in their practice, including diagrams illustrating the onset of labour, conceptual models cannot be represented in this concrete way. Pearson and Vaughan (1986) consider that conceptual models are in essence the same as the more physical models described above but may be described as descriptive pictures which represent practice: 'pictures composed of ideas and values and written down in a clear way' (Pearson and Vaughan, 1986, p. 2).

Four ideas, or concepts are central to all nursing models.

person
health
environment
nursing

All models of nursing can be analysed in terms of the emphasis given within each model to these elements or concepts (see for example Fawcett, 1984; Kershaw and Salvage, 1986; Fitzpatrick and Whall, 1989; Marriner-Tomey, 1989 and Moody, 1990). Each model gives greater or less weight to different elements. For example, the models of Florence Nightingale and Neuman emphasise the effects of the environment or society on health whereas for Rogers and Parse the person or individual is the central focus of their model. In addition to reflecting the views of individual nurse theorists, concern with the different elements reflects changes in society and nursing practice (Fitzpatrick and Whall, 1989).

Each of these models is, therefore, concerned with the person, the individual – what are the characteristics of the person and how does the person interrelate with the world? For example, King describes the person as follows: 'Human beings are viewed as open systems interacting with the environment, each exhibiting permeable boundaries permitting an exchange of matter, energy and information' (Gonot, 1989,

p. 273). While Orem's view of the person is described by Johnston (1989) as follows: 'In discussing the nature of the person, she considers the person as self-reliant and responsible for self-care and the wellbeing of dependents. Self-care is a requirement for persons. It is the capacity to reflect upon personal experience of self and environment, and the use of symbols (ideas, words), which distinguishes people from other species' (Johnston, 1989, p. 170).

Similarly, each model defines and elaborates a view of the concepts of environment (society), health and nursing practice. The particular philosophical orientation of the theorist, whether nurse or midwife, will determine the way in which they define the person, health, the environment and nursing practice. Pearson and Vaughan (1986) and Carveth (1987) summarise the main traditions on which models are based and which provide a means of classifying models. Systems models are based on systems theory in which closed and open systems are described. These models describe the process by which the individual seeks to maintain and adapt to or cope with changes in their external and internal environments. The models developed by Roy and Neuman are examples of systems models (see Chapter 7).

Another group of models is based on developmental theory. These models are centrally concerned with growth and change and the function of the nurse or midwife in facilitating this process. The inclusion in the activities of living model developed by Roper *et al.* (1985) of the concept of the life span is an example of the inclusion of developmental theory in a nursing model (see Chapter 7). A number of the models developed in relation to the care of the childbearing woman which are discussed in Chapter 6 are also concerned with the developmental process involved in becoming a mother and can therefore be classified as developmental models (Rubin, 1984; Mercer, 1986).

The models proposed by Rubin (1984) and Mercer (1986) are also based on symbolic interaction theory which is the theory which underpins the third group of nursing models. Symbolic interaction theory is concerned with the interaction between the individual and the environment and the interpretation that the individual puts on that interaction. It is concerned with the way that individuals construct their own roles (or ways of behaving) through the process of interaction with the environment, composed of other people, their expectations and the expectations implicit in the roles held by those individuals.

The symbolic interactionists operate on three premises: that the human being has a self; that human action is constructed by that self; that human action occurs within a social setting. (Field, 1983, p. 4)

These models put emphasis on understanding, empathising with the individual's view of their world and Reihl's model provides an example of this group of models (see Chapter 7). If the process of childbearing is viewed as a process in which the woman adopts and develops new understandings of herself, her relationships and her roles (as for example a daughter, friend and new mother) then it is clear why symbolic interaction is the basis of models concerned with attainment of the maternal role (Rubin, 1984; Mercer, 1986).

PARADIGMS

In much of the literature on models and theory building the four concepts identified above (person, health, environment and nursing) are described as metaparadigm concepts (Fawcett, 1984; Carveth, 1987; Moody, 1990). A paradigm is described as the world-view of a discipline: 'different disciplines often use different approaches to enquiry, according to the particular world-view, and hence *paradigm* they pursue' (Vaughan, 1992, p. 10). Robinson (1992) discusses the use of the term paradigm by the physicist Kuhn (1962) who used the term to describe a world-view held by a discipline, for example physicists held the world-view that the world was flat. Changes in the paradigm that the world was flat led to a huge shift or paradigm shift in the science of physics.

Vaughan (1992) describes three world-views, that of the natural sciences, that of naturalism and that of critical social theory. The first paradigm is that found in the basic sciences and knowledge is developed in this paradigm through positivism and experimentation. In the naturalism paradigm, knowledge is developed through observation of the natural world and attempts to explain the world through the experience of those in it. In the third paradigm, critical social theory, the individual is placed centrally in the development of theory which is developed by the reflection of the individual on their own world or their own practice. Vaughan (1992) notes that this paradigm and its approach to theory development has not been explored to any great extent in nursing as yet.

The term paradigm is also used by some authors (for example Moody, 1990) to describe conceptual models. Robinson (1992) argues that the models which have been developed in nursing do not constitute such paradigms, or world-views of nursing which are held in common by many nurses, and the description of paradigms given by Vaughan (1992) would support this analysis. Philosophies and conceptual models may be considered to be derived from paradigms so that a range of conceptual models may be derived from one paradigm (see

Table 2.1). For example, developmental models and systems models may all be described as emanating from the natural sciences world-view or paradigm, while symbolic interactionist models may be seen to be based on the naturalism world-view or paradigm. These conceptual models are based on and give rise to a range of theories about practice. The theories are comprised of a number of concepts which, when they are described in measurable terms, may be examined in practice. This examination in turn either strengthens or challenges the theory, the model, the philosophy and the paradigm.

The four concepts of person, health, environment and nursing are metaparadigm concepts in the sense that they appear to be held in common by all nurses as the central concepts underpinning practice. (It could perhaps be suggested that this apparently universal acceptance of these metaparadigm concepts may limit imagination and thinking about other concepts that might be important in nursing.) Any paradigm on which nursing is based should therefore contain an understanding of these concepts. In the following these metaparadigm concepts are referred to as concepts as they are considered in the context of conceptual models and theories rather than in the context of paradigms.

Table 2.1   *The relationship between paradigms, philosophies, models, theories and concepts*

Natural science paradigm

Philosophies

Conceptual models	
Developmental models, e.g.	Systems models, e.g.
Orem	Roy
Roper, Logan and Tierney	Neuman
A range of theories derived from each model	A range of theories derived from each model
A range of concepts that are related together in theories	A range of concepts that are related together in theories
Indicators of those concepts in practice	Indicators of those concepts in practice

CONCEPTS

From the description of conceptual models above, it is clear that the basic elements of a model are the concepts which are considered in that model. But what is a concept? One definition of 'concept' with which midwives will be familiar is the use of the word to mean: 'to conceive in the womb'(Simpson and Wiener, 1989, p. 653). However, this is not the meaning which is generally ascribed to the noun 'concept', used in the context of theory building. The phenomena which are brought together in a model are labelled concepts:

> These phenomena are classified into concepts, which are words bringing forth mental images of the properties of things. Concepts may be abstract ideas, such as adaptation and equilibrium, or concrete ones, such as table and chair. (Fawcett, 1992, p. 425)

The term concept is the label given to classes of ideas and things in the world and part of the process of learning involves the development of the understanding of concepts:

> Our world is filled with sets of objects, events and ideas that share some common quality while differing in other characteristics. An organism that learns to respond to the common quality of a given set has learned a concept. (Sills, 1972, p. 206)

This description indicates that a concept can be applied to an idea, an event or a group of objects. While the idea (concept) that other 'organisms' may recognise concepts as concepts may be questioned, this description shows that the individual's understanding of concepts develops through learning and observation. For example, a child learns through observation to identify the colour blue from the other properties of an object such as its weight or size (Sills, 1972; Chapman, 1985). Through observation and experience the individual develops a concept or idea of body-weight and the normal range of body-weight. The individual's mental picture, idea or concept of ideal body-weight will be influenced by the society within which they live, the social prestige given to those who are very heavy or very slim, access to food and health messages related to weight. Weight is a concrete concept. Other concepts are more abstract; for example, anxiety. Through experience and observation, an idea of the physical and psychological factors which combine together to produce the concept anxiety is developed. Concepts enable us to make sense of our world:

> Concepts are linguistic labels that selectively categorise elements of reality. Concepts are *mental images* that help organise the facts in

our world, thus enabling us to go about our daily activities in a more orderly fashion. Concepts are not real but invented to represent reality. (Moody, 1990, p. 148)

Concepts, this description suggests, are labels, not the things themselves. To observe or develop some aspect of a concept it has to be described or defined in more explicit, observable or measurable terms. Thompson *et al.* (1989), in a discussion of the process of theory building in nurse-midwifery, provide an example of this process. These authors identify six concepts which are: 'intended to promote the optimal health and wellbeing of women' (Thompson *et al.*, 1989, p. 124). These concepts are: safe; satisfying; respecting human dignity and self-determination; respecting cultural and ethnic diversity; family-centred; and health-promoting. Each of these concepts is defined and the components of the concept specified. Taking one example, 'satisfying', the definition and components identified within the definition are as follows:

Definition: actions that maximize congruence of woman's/family's preferences for care and expectations of outcomes with realities and actual health outcomes.

Components:
1. Identifies client preferences for pregnancy care
2. Helps mobilize resources throughout pregnancy to meet client preferences
3. Meets birth expectations of client and family when possible
4. Minimizes the negative aspects of health systems that affect the client
5. Applies current theory and research in order to provide the highest quality nurse-midwifery care

(Thompson *et al.*, 1989, p. 125)

Each of the components is then described in terms of an indicator of that component in practice. For example:

Components and indicators
1. Identifies client preferences for pregnancy or gynecologic care

Elicits and listens for client identification of preferences.
Tailors schedule of prenatal or gyn visits to needs and preferences of client.
Initiates information-seeking process about supplementary care that can be adapted to client preferences.

Identifies care options, including CNM or MD as the provider or
comanager.
Provides continuity of care including 24-hour access.

(Thompson *et al.*, 1989, p. 127)

This process of identification of concepts, definition and development of
indicators demonstrates the process by which model building, which involves the statement of the underlying philosophy of the midwife, the
naming of concepts and the description of relationships between concepts, the proposition of theories and measurement of the concepts in
practice, relates to the actual provision of care in practice. A model
which includes the concept, for example, of 'satisfying' as an aspect of
midwifery care will result in a different experience of care (if that model
is put into practice) than a model which does not include this concept.

THEORY

Conceptual models provide the broad framework of ideas about, for
example, midwifery care. These models are comprised of concepts.
Theories may be derived from conceptual models (through a process of
deductive theorising) or may be derived from observation (through a
process of inductive theorising). Theories contribute to the construction and testing of conceptual models and are more limited in scope
than models. Theories may (if they are predictive theories) suggest relationships between concepts in the form: 'if...then...' (Agyris and
Schön, 1974, p. 5). Using the example above, a theory could be suggested that: *if* the midwife listens to and identifies the woman's preferences *then* the woman will experience greater satisfaction in the care
that is provided.

Theory is essentially about providing explanations of events, actions
and phenomena. These explanations may arise through a process of
thinking, through a process of observation or through a combination of
thinking (incorporating prior knowledge) with observation. Once an explanation or theory has been expressed it can then be tested in practice
and through research. Theory which is predictive of practice is developed through a process which moves through descriptive or factor-
isolating theory, explanatory theory and predictive theory finally to
theory which is prescriptive (Dickoff and James, 1992) (see below).

The dictionary provides two definitions of the word 'theory':

A conception or mental scheme of something to be done, or of the
method of doing it; a systematic statement of rules or principles to be
followed;

A scheme or system of ideas or statements held as an explanation or account of a group of facts or phenomena; a hypothesis that has been confirmed or established by observation or experiment, and is propounded or accepted as accounting for the known facts; a statement of what are held to be the general laws, principles, or causes of something known or observed. (Simpson and Weiner, 1989, p. 902)

A theory is, therefore, a mental construct which seeks to clarify the relationships between facts and phenomena (between concepts). Moody (1990) cites Silva's (1981) definition of the term 'theory' which demonstrates the relationship between philosophy and theory:

The term *theory* refers to a set of logically inter-related statements of significance (concepts, propositions, definitions) that have been derived from philosophic beliefs or scientific data and from which questions or hypotheses can be deduced, tested and verified. (Silva, 1981, cited by Moody, 1990, p. 23)

Moody (1990) goes on to discuss the value and utility of theories in practice and research:

Theories are invented to assist us in describing, explaining, predicting and understanding phenomena of concern. In relation to research, theory helps us to interpret scientific findings in a meaningful and generalisable way. (Moody, 1990, p. 23).

In conclusion, Moody (1990) provides this succinct summary of the term:

A *theory* is a set of concepts or inter-related statements that may be tested empirically and serve to explain, describe or predict phenomena of interest to the discipline. (Moody, 1990, p. 57)

Concepts are described as the building blocks of theory (Chapman, 1985). Concepts brought together in theory provide an explanation of reality which may then be tested through observation in practice or through research. For example, in the 1920s the obstetrician Grantley Dick-Read brought together the concepts of fear and tension in a model to explain the pain that he had observed in women he was caring for in labour. The three concepts of fear, tension and pain were described by Dick-Read (1987) as follows:

Fear is a natural protective emotion without which few of us would survive. When through association or indoctrination there is fear of childbirth, resistant actions and reactions are brought to the mechanism of the organs of reproduction.

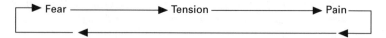

Figure 2.1   *The feedback relationship between fear, tension and pain*

This discord disturbs the harmony or polarity of muscle action, causing *tension*, which in turn gives rise to nervous impulses interpreted in the brain as *pain* (Dick-Read, 1987, p. 196).

This feedback relationship can be illustrated as shown in Figure 2.1. This theory of the relationship between fear, tension and pain was then addressed by Dick-Read through the provision of information on the process of labour through childbirth-preparation classes, books and other means.

The relationship between uncertainty, anxiety and pain has been extensively explored in the field of surgical nursing. Hayward (1975), for example, provides detailed definitions of these three concepts and describes the knowledge base from which these concepts were drawn. In a description of an experimental study of this theory, information is also provided of the ways in which these concepts were measured, including using a pain measure and recording administration of analgesia. This study found that people who had information about their surgery and what they should expect after the operation experienced less pain than people who did not have this information. In a study of information given to women in labour Kirkham (1989) has shown that, while women wanted information, there was no consistency in the information they were given and the midwives were constrained, in a number of ways, from giving information. Kirkham (1989) refers to Hayward's (1975) study and comments on the lack of application of these findings in care of the childbearing woman. Reference could also be made to the earlier work by Dick-Read (1987) on this theory which suggests an if...then... relationship between information and pain. Interestingly, Fawcett *et al.* (1993), coming from a different starting-point (the Roy Adaptation Model of Nursing) have more recently been studying the effects of information on adaptation to Caesarean birth (see Chapter 7) which is another contribution to the testing of the theory of the relationship between information and outcomes of midwifery care.

WHERE DOES THEORY COME FROM?

Having established some understanding of the terms theory, model and concept, this section will consider how theory is developed, and how knowledge is developed. Morse (1992) indicates that theory is developed from available information. This information may be available in the form of knowledge in a range of disciplines such as sociology, physiology or history or in the form of data or evidence from practice (empirical information). In the first case, theory is developed by deductive reasoning from the knowledge base that is already available, while in the second case, theory is developed inductively from the evidence. In both cases the theory can then be further tested, the theory developed and the knowledge base extended.

Deductive theory

In their book *Knowledge for Nursing Practice*, Robinson and Vaughan (1992) describe the variety of disciplines on which nursing knowledge is based and this applies to midwifery too (see Chapter 4). One example of the derivation of theory from other disciplines which is utilised in midwifery is provided by the range of theories about social deprivation and health which are derived from sociological theory. There is a great deal of evidence in the form of mortality and morbidity statistics that people in areas of deprivation experience poorer health than people who live in less deprived areas: this experience is part of the North–South divide in Britain and the South–North divide throughout the world. Theories have been propounded from many fields in relation to deprivation and health. In sociology, for example, the following theories have been deduced from the knowledge base of sociology to provide an explanation of the relationship between ill health and poverty:

- artifact theory – that the relationships are spurious and due to artifacts in data collection;
- social selection theory – that those in poor health cannot work and therefore move down into lower social classes;
- materialist theory – that material circumstances such as income and housing are the most important factors;
- cultural/behavioural theories – that class differences in health beliefs and behaviour have the most profound effects on health. (Jewson, 1993)

Each of these theories can be examined in relation to data to assess the extent to which the theory provides a true explanation of reality.

In the example above, theory is derived from one discipline. Theory may also be deduced or derived from a combination of disciplines. Shorney (1990) provides an example of the combination of knowledge from a large number of disciplines to provide a 'theory of healthy

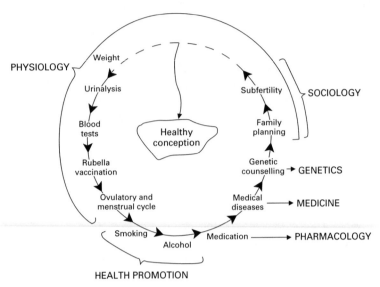

Figure 2.2   *Disciplines underpinning preconceptual care*

(Adapted from Shorney, *The Preconception Cycle of Care*, 1990,
Fig. 1.2, Reproduced with the permission of Macmillan Press Ltd)

conception' as shown in Figure 2.2. As this diagram shows, the elements or concepts which combine together to provide this 'theory of healthy conception' are derived from a number of disciplines and, in some cases, the concepts themselves may be derived from a variety of disciplines. For example, the concept of family planning is informed by pharmacology, physiology, education, psychology, sociology and other disciplines. Shorney's (1990) model of the 'preconception cycle of care' illustrates the application of theory to practice which is an everyday activity in midwifery care. Clark (1986) provides another illustration of this use of deductive theory in a discussion of the type of theory used in the giving of an injection including theory relating to the principles of aseptic technique, the pharmacology of the drug and the symbolic meaning the injection has for the patient and the nurse. Theory deduced from a wide range of knowledge areas therefore informs everyday practice situations and may be described as theory for or of practice. This is a use of theory which is familiar to every midwife.

Inductive theory

Theory may also be developed inductively from practice through the collection of evidence from practice. There are various approaches to this type of theory development including reflection-in-action, qualitative research and critical social theory. Schön (1983) describes reflection-in-action as follows:

> When someone reflects-in-action, he becomes a researcher in the practice context. He is not dependent on the categories of established theory and technique, but develops a new theory of the unique case. His inquiry is not limited to a deliberation about means which depends on a prior agreement about ends. (Schön, 1983, p. 68)

Qualitative research is aimed at understanding the views, feelings, attitudes and lives of a group of people through the collection of data about their experiences and lives through interviews, observation or other methods (Hakim, 1987). The information collected is then analysed and concepts in the data are identified and relationships between these concepts suggested. This process is illustrated in Kirkham's (1989) study in which she observed women in labour and identified, among other concepts, those of labelling, ward order and verbal asepsis in the data collected. This type of research then provides the basis for further deductive studies testing the relationships between the concepts which may then be related in a model of midwifery care and information-giving in labour.

In recent years the inductive approach to theory development based on reflection-in-action has received a great deal of attention in nursing due to the work of Benner and Wrubel (1989). Benner has pioneered the use of narrative descriptions of actual clinical practice as a means of describing and identifying the factors which constitute expert nursing practice. Alexander (1989) contrasts the approach taken by Benner and Wrubel (1989) (and others including Agyris and Schön (1974)) with the deductive (positivistic) approach to theory development:

> Utilising the scientific approach, one would look for lawlike relational statements to predict practice. Nevertheless, employing the qualitative methods in an interpretative approach, Benner describes expert nursing practice in many exemplars. Positivistic science takes an alternative approach by seeking formulas and models to apply. Her work seems to be hypotheses generating rather than hypotheses testing. Benner provides no universal 'how to' for nursing practice, but rather provides a methodology for uncovering and entering into the situated meaning of expert nursing care. (Alexander, 1989, p. 196)

Using this method, nurses describe clinical practice events and use these as the starting-point for ideas (theories) about clinical interventions which may be more or less helpful. These theories can then be tried out in subsequent clinical situations. The basis of this approach is an attempt to elucidate the theories-in-use that are used by the skilled nurse or midwife and it is based on the view that formal (deductive) theory cannot provide the total explanation for an event in clinical practice. Expert clinical practice is an amalgam of deductive theory with observation, interpretation and experimentation by the practitioner in the field of practice. Agyris and Schön (1974) illustrate this with the example of grammar and speech. Few people can describe the theories of grammar but everyone demonstrates their own interpretation of these theories in their use of grammar, their theory-in-use of grammar. Alexander (1989) describes this process in Benner's work:

> Benner stated that theory is crucial in order to form the right questions to ask in a clinical situation; theory directs the practitioner in looking for problems and anticipating care needs. There is always more to any situation than theory predicts. The skilled practice of nursing exceeds the bounds of formal theory. Concrete experience provides the learning about the exceptions and shades of meaning in a situation. The knowledge embedded in practice discovers and interprets theory, precedes or extends theory, and synthesises and adapts theory in caring nursing practice. (Alexander, 1989, p. 193)

Midwives may have sympathy with this description of the inductive development of theory. Much of the antagonism to the exploration of the use of theory in practice, it is suggested, may be based on the experience of the expert practitioner that much deductive theory, derived from conceptual models, is too simplistic and does not provide an adequate explanation for the complexity of midwifery care. Benner and Wrubel (1989) provide a challenge to all clinical practitioners, including midwives, to describe and tease out from descriptions of clinical care those factors which are significant in that care. Descriptions of these factors and the relationships between the factors (hypotheses) can then be tested in other clinical situations and practice theory developed. However, exploration of this type of theory is not easy and midwives, in common with other clinical practitioners may prefer to keep away from the exploration and misunderstandings of the 'swampy lowlands':

> In the varied topography of professional practice, there is a high hard ground where practitioners can make effective use of research-based theory and technique, and there is a swampy lowland where situations are confusing 'messes' incapable of technical solution. (Schön, 1983, p. 42).

Schön (1983) suggests that the problems encompassed in the 'messes' are of particular concern to the person affected but may be given less attention by professionals as the problems are not amenable to treatment or alteration using the theories and techniques available to the professional. There may indeed be different types of professional. Schön (1983) suggests that those who choose to work in the swampy lowlands 'deliberately involve themselves in messy but crucially important problems and, when asked to describe their methods of inquiry they speak of experience, trial and error, intuition and muddling through' (Schön, 1983, p. 43). While:

> Other professionals opt for the high ground. Hungry for technical rigour, devoted to an image of solid professional competence, or fearful of entering a world in which they feel they do not know what they are doing, they choose to confine themselves to narrowly technical practice. (Schön, 1983, p. 43)

Benner (1984) provides a means of demonstrating, exploring and developing some understanding of the 'swampy lowlands' of practice as well as the 'high hard ground'.

One danger that needs to be guarded against in the exploration of the 'swampy lowlands' is that creative practice may be assumed to rest on experience alone rather than being an expression of the interpretation of knowledge and deductive theory from a range of disciplines which is transformed by the skilled practitioner in their theory-in-use, as Benner and Wrubel (1989) acknowledge. Powell (1989) expressed concern about nursing care when she observed that: 'The nurse would try various methods of assisting the patient, often producing helpful results but in a time consuming and essentially unthinking way' (Powell, 1989, p. 829). This author argues for the careful combination of theory (deductive theory) with theorising from practice (inductive theory):

> The need is, therefore, for theories of practice, based on sound theories-in-use, where an essential ingredient would appear to be an in-depth knowledge base in both nursing theory and contributing disciplines. Should this be of poor quality, the theories of practice will be ineffective in terms of patient care and use of resources, human and material. (Powell, 1989, p. 830).

Combining deductive and inductive theory

There is an argument within the nursing literature that more weight has been given in the past to models, theory and knowledge derived from disciplines outside nursing than to theory which has now been developed from practice. The same arguments could possibly apply in midwifery although the debate about the use of models and theory in midwifery is only just gathering momentum. In the debate in nursing and other fields, such as education, it appears that, to make the point more strongly for the value of practice theory, advocates of experiential learning have decried the value of knowledge from sources other than the experiential, practice base, as discussed above. This leads to the danger that practitioners may have inadequate knowledge, for example, of physiology or psychology, which limits their ability to be creative in practice situations in the way envisaged in Benner's (1984) model of the expert practitioner.

Boud *et al.* (1985) epitomise this approach in their description of experiential learning as freeing people 'from the drudgery of organising complicated bodies of knowledge' (p. 43). Myths and other messages about learning support this denial. For example, a poster depicts Einstein with the quotation: 'Imagination is more important than knowledge', implying that we, who have little or no knowledge, can achieve as much as Einstein through the use of our imaginations! Newton provides the most ironic example of this type of myth. Newton was an architect of the deductive, scientific method but has been portrayed as one of the chief exponents of experiential learning – through the experience of an apple falling on his head, he discovered gravity!

The reality of this discovery is in fact very different. Newton spent many years studying prior to developing his theory about gravity. In 1661, when he was 19, he went to university, where he studied the official curriculum of Greek philosophy and his own unofficial curriculum of seventeenth-century philosophers, scientists and mathematicians. This knowledge provided the foundation for his discoveries and theories in mathematics, dynamics, optics and many other fields (Fauvel *et al.*, 1989).

The amount of work involved in studying in the way that Newton studied is enormous. Is it for this reason that the myth of the apple is so strong? It is much more comfortable to think that we might one day sit under an apple tree (or care for a woman during the childbearing process) and discover one of the secrets of the universe than that we might have to spend many years absorbing the accumulated knowledge of our forebears and then examine our own experience in the light of that knowledge. However, subject areas are not called disciplines for no reason. If each of us had to reinvent the wheel would we have made a bicycle let alone a car by the end of our lives?

Creative midwifery practice, it is therefore argued, must be dependent on the utilisation of theory derived from a range of disciplines in combination with practice theories.

Levels of theory

In the preceding discussion the basic form of a theory has been described as a means of stating relationships between concepts. Theories may be described according to their scope. Although different terms are used by different authors the following are commonly described: microtheories, middle-range theories and grand theory, paradigms and meta-theory. In addition, Moody (1990) identifies practice theory as a separate category. Practice theory, as discussed above, is derived from direct observation and reflection on practice, from an inductive process. Both microtheories and middle-range theories may be derived, at least in part, from such a process. Thus it may be more useful to consider practice theory as one type of microtheory, other types of microtheory being derived from deductive reasoning.

Microtheories are described by Keck (1989) as:

> the least complex [theories]. They contain the least complex concepts and refer to scientific, easily defined phenomena. They are narrow in scope because they attempt to explain a small aspect of reality. They are primarily composed of enumerative or associative concepts. (Keck, 1989, pp. 21–2).

Middle-range theories are theories at the next level of complexity (Marriner-Tomey, 1989). Moody (1990) cites Merton's (1968) definition of middle-range theories: 'as those that examine a portion of reality and identify a few key variables: Propositions are clearly formulated and testable hypotheses can be derived.' (Moody, 1990, p. 55).

Moody (1990) comments that middle-range theories are often developed by qualitative or ethnographic studies in which data is collected about an area of practice or experience. Variables or concepts are identified in the data and suggestions (propositions or hypotheses) are then made about the relationship between the different variables. These relationships can then be tested by further research. Lehrman (1989) describes the model she has developed, the Nurse-Midwifery Practice Model, as a middle-range theory and describes research aimed at testing relationships between concepts in part of the model which is concerned with care in labour (Lehrman, 1988) (see Chapter 6).

Grand theories are 'the most complex and broadest in scope. They attempt to explain areas in a discipline. They are composed of summative concepts and incorporate numerous narrow range theories' (Keck, 1989, p. 22).

The final level of theory is meta-theory which is 'the analysis of theory or theorising about theory in a discipline' (Moody, 1990, p. 55). Meta-analysis is a method made familiar in midwifery practice through the work of Enkin *et al.* (1991) who, with their colleagues, have brought together a huge amount of research in areas of pregnancy and childbirth. This research has been combined and analysed to produce information about the most effective methods of care. In the same way theories may be analysed and considered in relation to the concepts included in the theories, the relevance of the theories to the discipline, the strength of relationships between concepts, and so on.

Types of theory

Four types of theory have been described by Dickoff and James (1992), two philosophers who have worked closely with nurses for many years, in their classic paper: 'A Theory of Theories: A Position Paper' written in 1968. Theories may either describe, explain, predict, produce or shape reality. Moody (1990) summarises these four levels of theory:

(1) factor-isolating theories: observing, describing and naming concepts
(2) factor-relating theories: relating named concepts to one another
(3) situation-relating theories: inter-relationships among concepts or propositions
(4) situation-producing theories: prescribing activities necessary to reach defined goals (also known as prescriptive theories). (Moody, 1990, p. 54)

The first level of theory identifies and describes or names concepts. Dickoff *et al.* (1992a) describe this as naming theory and point out that, if concepts have not been named, further levels of theory development are impossible. Much of midwifery and nursing research is descriptive and aimed at this first level of theory: naming the concepts in midwifery. The process of identifying the concepts in midwifery is addressed in Chapters 5, 6 and 7.

Factor-relating theories suggest interrelationships between concepts. Such theories are often the outcome of qualitative research in which factors have been named and then relationships between them suggested. Situation-relating theories are the third level of theory and are predictive theories. Such theories predict that if one factor or variable is altered there will be an change in one or more other variables.

The fourth level of theory is described as situation-producing theory and is aimed at bringing about change:

> predictive theory says if A happens then B happens; prescriptive or situation-producing theory says B is among the things conceived as appropriate to bring into being and so here is how to bring about A, or here is how to facilitate A's production of B, and so on. (Dickoff *et al.*, 1992a, pp. 477–8)

Dickoff *et al.* (1992b) concluded in 1968 that none of the existing theories of nursing met their criteria for a fourth level situation-producing theory. There are, however, multiple theories of the first, second and third types. In fact, there are so many theories and models of and for nursing that Whall (1989) has argued that, rather than develop new theories, nurses should be developing and refining those already available. This is a point that midwives may need to consider as theoretical development proceeds: are there ways of networking and sharing ideas about theory development which may be more useful for care of the childbearing woman than the development of multiple theories? The argument in opposition to this is that each human being and their circumstance is unique and therefore multiple theories are needed. Might there be, however, concepts which would be inherent in any model of midwifery practice?

CONCEPTS BASIC TO MIDWIFERY

Earlier, the four concepts which are described as being basic to all models of nursing were described: the person, health, the environment and nursing. For midwifery these elements could be:

> person (the woman, child, partner and others)
> health
> environment
> midwifery

Theories or models of or for midwifery practice would therefore contain these concepts. Later parts of this book will consider theory used in midwifery practice and the extent to which these concepts are elaborated in these theories.

But prior to examining these theories it may be worth considering the following questions relating to these concepts. How do I think about people: the woman and families I care for? How do I think about

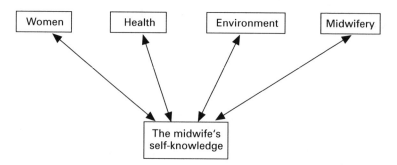

Figure 2.3   *Concepts central to midwifery care*

health? How do I think about the environment and society? How do I
think about midwifery practice? Thinking about these areas brings together knowledge from other disciplines such as psychology, our own
experiences as women (or men) and our values and attitudes, developed throughout our lives. And it is this element, it is suggested, that is
missing from the characterisation of models as being concerned with
the concepts of person, health, environment and midwifery. A fifth
element is the personal or self-knowledge discussed earlier (Carper,
1992). It may be suggested that any model of midwifery should also
include the concept of personal knowledge which underpins the other
concepts as shown in Figure 2.3.

A conceptual model of midwifery would provide a picture of midwifery practice and care and help provide answers to questions about
what constitutes midwifery practice.

In summary, conceptual models provide an abstract picture of the
thinking of one or more people about some aspect of the world; in the
case of midwifery, midwifery care. Theories are formulated from an
understanding of the relationships between concepts and may be tested
through observation and other forms of research. Models and theories
are mental constructs and this must always be remembered. They are
mental constructs or images developed to provide greater understanding of events in the physical, psychological or social worlds. Models
and theories are not concrete objects and are intended to be tested,
modified or abandoned in the light of new evidence. For example, the
theory that the world was flat was abandoned (by most people) when
new evidence was discovered. As an advertisement for beer which
shows a picture of a flat earth puts it: 'When you know what's what and
what's not.' Similarly, the model of faecal contamination at delivery
held until very recently was abandoned in the light of research findings
and a new model substituted (Romney and White, 1984).

Morse (1992) has cautioned against the danger of 'believing in theories':

> Theories, theoretical frameworks, and models have been taught to students as *facts*, as correct and as dogma. Students have been examined on the material, graded and instructed to somehow use these theories in practice. What they have *not* been taught is that theories are only *tools*; that theories are means for organising data, for making sense of and explaining reality, so that confusion is rendered comprehensible and predictable. Students have not been taught that theories are merely someone's best guess about the nature of reality – given the available information – and as such, they must be tested, modified, and tested again. (Morse, 1992, p. 259)

THEORIES AND MODELS FOR WHAT?

Implicit in this chapter has been the assumption that the identification of concepts underlying midwifery practice, the examination of theory and development of models, either deductively or inductively, has a value for practice, education and research. Hughes (1988) has argued that midwifery should not be practised 'in an erratic and whimsical way' (p. 2) but is concerned that nursing models do not appear to offer a great deal to midwifery practice which is largely constrained, she argues, by organisational factors: 'How can "models" challenge the constraints which thwart good midwifery now?' (Hughes, 1988, p. 2). Rothman (1983) illustrates this process in a description of the different models of labour and delivery held by nurse-midwives. The effect of 'the system' on the conduct of labour and the conflicts caused for these practitioners of normal midwifery in a medical context is very clear. However, Aaronson (1987) has shown that the care provided by nurse-midwives and obstetricians working within the same system is perceived as being qualitatively different by women. Women, with similar demographic characteristics, perceived the care they received from obstetricians and nurse-midwives to be different in terms of the different health practitioners' feelings about certain health behaviours and their supportiveness to the women. It can be suggested that these differences reflect the differences in the models of care held by the nurse-midwives and the obstetricians.

It is the contention of this book that personal models of care do affect practice and therefore need to be explored. However, the history and present experience of midwifery demonstrate the influence of the organisational culture on practice and it is for this reason that these issues are addressed in Chapter 3. It is suggested that an understanding of the personal factors, the organisational factors and the societal factors which affect midwifery practice is needed so that midwifery care may be developed to enable all women to experience midwifery care which is supportive and personal.

Summary

In this chapter the main tools that are used in thinking about practice have been discussed. Thinking about practice involves the consideration of underlying beliefs and values expressed in paradigms and philosophies. It involves the identification of concepts that are central to midwifery and which, when combined together in theories and conceptual models, provide ways in which midwifery care may be understood, tested and examined. This understanding also enables the planning of change and introduction of new models in ways which recognise the existence of the different models held by midwives and other health care practitioners providing maternity care.

Activities

Using the material in this chapter, review the chapter by considering the following activities in relation to your own practice.

1 Describe a practical care activity that you have been involved in recently and describe the different types of knowledge which informed your care.
2 With reference to the activity described in 1 above identify the midwifery science, the art of midwifery, your personal knowledge of yourself and the ethical knowledge which was included in this care.
3 What are the beliefs and values you hold about midwifery practice?
4 Describe the meaning of 'conceptual model' and identify some conceptual models with which you are familiar or which you use in your practice.
5 Describe the concepts that you consider are central to your conceptual model of care (with reference to 3 above).
6 Consider the four concepts identified as possibly central to midwifery models and consider: How do I think about people: the woman and families I care for? How do I think about health? How do I think about the environment and society? How do I think about midwifery practice?
7 Describe your conceptual model of midwifery care.

8 Considering the paradigms discussed above, on which paradigm do you consider your view of the world is based?

9 Identify two theories that you use in your practice, one deductive theory and one inductive theory. Describe the concepts that make up those theories.

10 How would you measure the concepts identified in 5 above in practice?

11 How would you categorise the theories you identified in 9?

12 What are your views of the importance of the self of the midwife in midwifery care? In what ways do you find support in undertaking midwifery care?

CHAPTER THREE

The context of midwifery care

Whether the change is sought or resisted, and happens by chance or design; whether we look at it from the standpoint of reformers or those they manipulate, of individuals or institutions, the response is characteristically ambivalent. The will to adapt to change has to overcome an impulse to restore the past which is equally universal. What becomes of a widow, a displaced family, a new organisation or a new way of business depends on how these conflicting impulses work themselves out, within each person and his or her relationships. (Marris, 1986, p. 5)

INTRODUCTION

As noted in Chapter 1, the organisational context of midwifery practice has a significant impact on midwifery care, midwifery action. It is the purpose of this chapter to consider some of the effects of the organisational context within which midwives practice, on midwifery care, midwifery action. The discussion in Chapters 1 and 2 has shown that the provision of midwifery care is not an activity which is value-free. The beliefs and values held by the individual midwife will have a profound affect on the way that the midwife thinks about women, pregnancy, the role of the midwife and the type of care that the midwife should provide.

Midwives rarely work individually or in independent practice but work, in Britain, largely in the context of the National Health Service (NHS). Even those midwives who work independently in Britain, who numbered only 66 in 1993 (Independent Midwives Association, 1993), work in partnership with midwives and others working within the NHS. The NHS is a huge organisation that can be seen to comprise many smaller organisations including hospitals, general practitioner units, midwife-led units and community units. Individual midwives hold different attitudes and beliefs about the care of the childbearing woman.

In the same way, organisations will have different values and aims which will be found in formal statements, for example in published philosophies, and informal values, aims and purposes that will be demonstrated in the structures and activities of the organisation.

This chapter explores the interrelationship of the models held by those working in an organisation with the models held in society and the models held by the organisation. The action approach to organisations is discussed as a means of understanding the complex interrelationships between society, organisations, practitioners, women and the care of the childbearing woman (Silverman, 1970). Following a consideration of the issues involved in the process of change, the organisation of maternity services in the Netherlands is presented as an example of the different type of care achieved within a society which holds an alternative view of pregnancy and childbirth.

The point should perhaps be made here that 'the organisation' is used here as a short-hand term. An organisation is not a thing but is made up of many people fulfilling many role descriptions and working towards ends that have been decided by people working within the organisation. Silverman (1970) identifies the process of describing an organisation as a thing as reification:

> We reify society if we regard it as having an existence which is separate from and above the actions of men: social roles and institutions exist only as an expression of the meanings which men attach to the world. (Silverman, 1970, p. 134)

In the following discussion, the danger of reification is acknowledged and the term 'the organisation' is used as a means to aid communication and does not imply that organisations have a life of their own.

INSTITUTIONS AND MIDWIFERY CARE

'Midwifery care is aimed at meeting the needs of women, their babies and their families' – or is it? This routine statement of the purpose of midwifery care provides one view of practice. Other views suggest that much of midwifery work is aimed at meeting the needs of obstetricians, other midwives (for example midwifery managers), the needs of individual midwives themselves and the needs of the organisation for the smooth running of the organisation. In your everyday practice, whose needs predominate in the type of care you are able to provide? Do you think that the context, the place in which you work, has any effect on the type of care you are able to provide to individual women?

Prior to the establishment of the NHS the majority of women were cared for in their own community, in their own home by the local midwife who worked in cooperation with the local general practitioner (Lewis, 1980; Roberts, 1984; Leap and Hunter, 1993). Leap and Hunter (1993), in their interviews with midwives who were practising in the 1920s onwards, provide descriptions of the community-based nature of the midwife's work and the autonomy that she had. In this situation the care that the woman received would be very dependent on the individual practice of the midwife, her knowledge and models of practice.

Throughout the twentieth century, care of the childbearing woman has moved from the community to the hospital setting. This move provided women with access to different forms of pain relief and other facilities, and has had benefits and consequences for midwives and obstetricians. Since the establishment of the NHS in 1948, there has been an acceleration in the movement of the care of women from the community into the institutional, hospital setting (Currell, 1990; Wraight *et al.*, 1993). Over 98 per cent of births take place in hospitals and a large proportion of antenatal care occurs in hospitals.

Stacy (1988) describes the growth in the power of the medical profession since the seventeenth century and the growth of hospitals as places where doctors could hold positions of authority and power. This development was also found in obstetrics, where the influence of medical men and man-midwives grew throughout the eighteenth and nineteenth centuries (Towler and Bramall, 1986; Donnison, 1988). Both Towler and Bramall (1986) and Donnison (1988) provide graphic descriptions of the takeover of care of the childbearing woman from midwives by male doctors. Towler and Bramall (1986) succinctly summarise the two facets of this takeover: gender and status/education in a discussion of the 'Master of British Midwifery' William Smellie:

> His skills would be difficult to equal, but despite this and regardless of their ability (or lack of it), all doctor practitioners were subsequently seen as 'superior' to midwives, purely on the grounds of their gender and education, which endowed them with a higher social status. (Towler and Bramall, 1986, pp. 103–4)

The hospitalisation of birth can be seen as part of the wider push by the medical profession for the hospitalisation of all health care. The hospitalisation of birth led to greater involvement of obstetricians in birth and the greater use of technology (Donnison, 1988; Wraight *et al.*, 1993). Government reports during the 1950s to the 1980s, as Currell (1990) describes, supported the hospitalisation of birth. For the midwife, hospitalisation of childbirth has had huge consequences for practice and for the place in which the midwife undertakes most care activities: traditionally the home, now the hospital. Benoit (1992) and Leap and Hunter (1993) warn against an over-romantic view of home-based midwifery practice in the past but, whatever the standards of that practice were, the change in place of practice has certainly occurred. From being the midwife for a community, caring for women and their daughters often over many years, the majority of midwives now work in hospitals. In hospitals care is divided between different departments, antenatal, postnatal and labour, and midwives' skills are thus divided and continuity of carer is difficult to achieve (Robinson *et al.*, 1983; Wraight *et al.*, 1993).

The effect of the organisational setting is illustrated by Benoit (1987; 1989). Benoit, using a number of criteria which relate to the description of a profession, describes midwives working in different settings in Newfoundland and Labrador as pre-professionals, technocrats and professionals. The pre-professionals are the granny midwives, who lack formal education and midwives working in isolated situations where they lack colleague support. The professional midwives she describes are those that used to work in cottage hospitals who had a high degree of autonomy of practice:

> The work autonomy of the cottage midwives was multifaceted. Full-fledged maternity attendants of pregnant women throughout their reproductive cycle, they occupied the strategic first point of entry for clients seeking health care. Cottage midwives followed the progress of pregnancies, monitored clients' labour process and delivered the baby, calling in a doctor only in cases of anticipated abnormality. (Benoit, 1987, pp. 251–2)

The midwives interviewed by Benoit (1987), and whom she describes as technocrats, were those midwives (the majority of midwives) working in large-scale organisations (in this part of Canada referred to as regional centres). Benoit describes this midwife as being controlled by hospital administrators, being involved in only a part of the care of the pregnant woman, not being able to exercise all her skills, lacking colleagueship with other midwives and acting as a doctor's handmaiden in a bureaucratic setting where doctors have responsibility for the normal, as well as the abnormal, aspects of childbearing. The following description will ring hollow bells for many midwives:

> She finds herself under the watchful eye of a hospital administration employing the latest bureaucratic management strategies to control work pace in an effort to remain within budgetary limits. She wants

to manage the 'whole show', using her own discretion in calling upon neighbouring occupations, yet finds herself in competition with doctors, nurses and even students in the performance of maternity tasks. Since physicians have usurped both normal and abnormal deliveries, the regional midwife has essentially become a doctor's handmaiden. Prior to the client's delivery she is pushed from centre stage and the medical experts (sometimes even hospital clerks) perform the 'high-powered stuff'. This situation leads to increasing estrangement between the regional midwife and the pregnant woman.... (Benoit, 1987, pp. 244–5)

Benoit (1992) has also compared the working situations of midwives in Sweden and the Netherlands with those of the midwives in Labrador and Newfoundland. In Sweden, women with uncomplicated pregnancies are cared for in local mothercare centres, small maternity units which are run by midwives who are employed by the state. Benoit (1992) describes these midwives as having considerable autonomy while having financial security. In the Netherlands midwives are independent contractors who are paid a fee by the insurance system for the care they provide. Benoit (1992) suggests that, while these midwives also have considerable autonomy, their care is affected by the financial pressures exerted by this system. She comments that the midwives in the Netherlands are 'caught in the age-old paradox affecting all non-salaried service practitioners: they need to run a successful business while also providing family-centered care to their homebirth clients' (Benoit, 1992, p. 211).

Additional evidence of the effect of the setting on practice is provided by the work of Garcia *et al.* (1987) and Garforth and Garcia (1987) who have demonstrated the continued use of perineal shaving and enemas when women are admitted in labour. The rates of use vary considerably between units in different health districts, supporting the conclusion that the rationales for these forms of intervention were based on hospital policies rather than the individual needs of the women. Barclay *et al.* (1989) have examined the place of midwifery care from the perspective of economics and identify: 'Women's business as big business' (p. 126). These authors also comment on the role of the midwife, identifying professionalisation rather than the place of activity as a factor which dehumanises birth:

> The midwife frequently acts as the agent that helps transform birth into a medical ritual. It is not surprising that this occurs, as the notion of midwife has changed from one of women with women, to a professional role in itself. (Barclay *et al.*, 1989, p. 123)

It may perhaps be suggested that the midwife's role, that Barclay *et al.* (1989) describe, has developed in this way due to the organisational setting and the relationship between midwifery practice and obstetrics. The evidence seems to suggest that midwives working in units that are led by midwives or general practitioners provide care which is perceived by women to be highly satisfactory (NHS Management Executive, 1993).

These examples indicate that the context within which midwives practice does have consequences for the work of the midwife and for the care that the midwife is able to provide. The structures of large organisations, such as hospitals, and of small organisations, such as small midwifery-led units or independent practices, both have consequences for midwifery care.

Concern has been expressed for a considerable time about the organisational context of maternity services and the consequences for the women of care in large organisations. Sullivan and Weitz (1988) identify Grantley Dick-Read as the person who made the first significant impact on medically dominated childbirth practices in the USA in the 1940s. Dick-Read argued for attention to be given to the natural process of birth, the psychological needs of women and the need for women and their partners to understand the process of birth. It is salutary to reflect that Dick-Read's first book on the subject of natural childbirth was published over 60 years ago (in 1933).

Donnison (1988) describes the concerns of consumer groups, which increased during the 1970s and 1980s as intervention in childbirth increased, and identifies the publication of *Having a Baby in Europe* (World Health Organization, 1985a) as the turning-point for those who were arguing for a more 'low-tech' approach to birth. Since the publication of this report there has been extensive debate in Britain about the structure and organisation of childbirth services which has resulted in the publication of the Winterton Report (House of Commons Health Committee, 1992) and the Expert Committee Report (Department of Health, 1993a and 1993b).

These reports highlight the problem areas within the current organisations in which most women receive care during pregnancy, labour and the postnatal period. The identification of the three main areas of concern – 'continuity', 'choice' and 'control' – indicates that the present systems do not help the woman to experience continuity, exercise choice, or control what happens to her during her care. Factors which inhibit the achievement of the three Cs can be illustrated with a few examples from the objectives and recommendations in these reports. Continuity of care, it is suggested, suffers from the exercise of professional power:

We further believe that the discussions we have heard about the case for providing continuity of care and the enabling of women to control their own pregnancies and deliveries have been far too heavily influenced by territorial disputes between the professionals concerned for control of the women whom they are supposed to be helping. (House of Commons Health Committee, 1992, p. xxxix)

Lack of involvement of women at all stages in the planning and monitoring of services reduces their control of the services:

Users of maternity services should be actively involved in planning and reviewing services. The lay representation must reflect the ethnic, cultural and social mix of the local population. A Maternity Services Liaison Committee should be established within every district health authority. (Department of Health, 1993a, p. 47)

And lack of use of midwives' skills limits choice:

The part which the midwife plays in maternity care should make full use of all her skills and knowledge, and reflect the full role for which she has been trained. (Department of Health, 1993a, p. 39)

We recommend that the development of midwifery-managed units, combined with effective continuity of midwifery care between the community and hospital, should be pursued by all DHAs. (House of Commons Health Committee, 1992, p. lxix)

These, and many of the other recommendations will require, in some cases, radical rethinking of the organisation of care. Current service patterns have grown in ways that meet needs as perceived by the powerful professional groups within maternity service provision. There is evidence that this radical rethinking is starting. A consultant obstetrician, Mr Malcolm Pearce, has been reported as calling for half of all consultant obstetricians to be sacked and for midwives to undertake the majority of care. In conjunction with this suggestion he has proposed the creation of a new type of consultant in a super-speciality of fetal-medicine who would care for women who were particularly at-risk (Pallot, 1993, p. 4).

It has been suggested that the hospitalisation of birth occurred in parallel to the general increase in the importance of hospitals as places of medical influence. The influence of the medical model grew in society and the growth of hospitals was one of the manifestations of influence of this model (see Chapter 4). It is evident that there is a whole range of factors which influence change in society and in organisations. Consumer groups, professional bodies and government reports may be identified in the above discussion as some of the influences for change and wider influences may also be identified. A reading of the Expert Committee Report (Department of Health, 1993a) demonstrates the influence of the Health for All Model on the recommendations (see Chapter 4). For example, the report recommends that care should be based in the community; it should be appropriate, accessible, effective and efficient and women should be involved in decisions about their care and in planning services (participation). Concern has been expressed about the medicalisation of childbirth for at least 60 years but it is only since 1985 that policymakers in Europe have reacted to these concerns in any way other than to reinforce the medical model (World Health Organization, 1985a). Now, with the use of an alternative model, policymakers are seeking to influence the organisation of health services in general and maternity services in particular. How will organisations respond to these efforts? What are the factors within organisations which influence the care that they provide? The next section goes on to consider some of these factors.

TYPES OF ORGANISATIONS

In a discussion of the different types of organisations Handy (1976) identifies over 60 variables or concepts that may be important for an understanding of the effectiveness of an organisation. These variables relate to leadership styles, group relations, the physical environment, personal characteristics of the work force and other factors. An enormous range of factors thus affects the output of an organisation, the care or action.

External factors which affect midwifery care have been described by DeVries (1993), who considers the impact of external, societal level factors, that is, factors outside the organisation, on midwifery practice. These factors are multi-faceted and at the societal level, he suggests, there are four factors or concepts which are crucial in an understanding of the practice of midwifery: geography; technology; the structure of society; and culture. Geography affects, among other things, the organisation of services and the support available to individual midwives who may be working in isolated situations. Technology, ranging from the mat and razor blade used by the traditional birth attendant to the sophisticated machinery used in many hospitals, considerably affects the practice and content of care. The structure of society which includes 'occupational structures and the arrangements between medical organisations and other institutions – political, legal, economic, religious, educational' (DeVries, 1993, p. 133) also has a significant impact on care while an understanding of the cultural context is vital to an understanding of the birth practices and care in any society. These factors are interrelated and it is this interrelationship which Handy (1976) considers contributes to the effectiveness of an organisation. Organisations are clearly complex bodies and many attempts have been made to explain the workings of organisations to enhance their effectiveness and to assist in the process of change.

All aspects of life are dominated by organisations. The growth of organisations was accelerated by the Industrial Revolution and development of technology. This can be seen in the field of midwifery, with the development of forceps, and more recent technological developments which increase the instrumental monitoring of pregnancy and reduce dependence on the skills of midwives (DeVries, 1993). Russell (1930), quoted in Khan *et al.* (1964) suggested growth of organisations occurred as 'mankind decided that it would submit to monotony and tedium in order to diminish the risk of starvation' (Khan *et al.*, 1964, p. 4). Or, in the case of childbirth, to reduce the risks inherent in childbearing through the adoption of the restrictive medical model which was considered as the model able to provide some control of physical risk.

Traditional organisational theory is concerned with the study of formal organisations as opposed to social organisations (Silverman, 1970). Formal organisations are differentiated from social organisations by the presence of goals and a formal structure to achieve goals. Weber (1957) described formal organisations, or bureaucracies, as organisations which demonstrated hierarchical authority, division of labour into defined tasks, systematic rules and impersonality (Goss, 1963; Dunkerley, 1972). Weber described an ideal type (a mental picture or conceptual model) to assist in the understanding of the ways in which organisations go about their business and achieve their ends. This ideal type suggests relationships between concepts such as power and role position which can then be tested through the observation and the collection of data in different organisations. Testing of the ideal type model of bureaucracy in this way has shown that different organisations are closer to the conceptual model than others. Studies of hospitals as organisations have shown that there are several hierarchies of authority rather than one, and the content of work may vary according to the grade of staff available rather than being limited to one grade, one role position, as suggested in the ideal type (Davies and Francis, 1976).

Inadequacies in the bureaucratic model have led to the development of alternative models to explain the activities and outcomes of health care and other organisations. A significant feature of health care organisations is the role that professional groups play within them and this has resulted in models of hospitals as professional organisations (Davies and Francis, 1976). Davies and Francis (1976) describe three such models. In the first, the professional organisation of work is characterised as requiring a different division of labour, training and means of control than that found in bureaucracies. The second model is derived from the work of Freidson (1970; 1975) who described professions as being in relationships of dominance and domination. This model focuses on the power that one profession, in Freidson's case the medical profession, exercises over other professions and occupational groups within an organisation (Hugman, 1991). This model describes professionals as having great control over their actions and shedding routine work to other occupational groups. The third model takes as its central concern the relationship between professional groups and is termed the negotiated order model. The hospital is viewed as an arena within which negotiation constantly takes place between different professional groups, who hold different aims and ideologies, to secure positions of power and influence (Strauss *et al.*, 1964; Davies and Francis, 1976).

Handy (1976) provides another way of looking at and representing organisations, through consideration of the culture of the organisation. He describes four types of organisation: the power culture; the role culture; the task culture; and the person culture. The power culture he describes as a spider's web with a powerful individual in the centre of the web controlling the activities in the organisation. Family businesses and some types of teams, for example medical teams, may be described as operating within a power culture. As Handy (1976) comments: 'If this culture had a patron god it would be Zeus, the powerful head of the Gods of Ancient Greece who ruled by whim and impulse, by thunderbolt and shower of gold from Mount Olympus' (Handy, 1976, p. 178).

Role cultures are the bureaucracy culture described above. These organisations are characterised by departments, roles and job descriptions: 'the role, or job description, is often more important than the individual who fills it' (Handy, 1976, p. 180). The structure is pictured by Handy as a Greek temple where the organisation is supported by firm pillars in the form of the different departments that make up the organisation. Handy suggests that Apollo, the god of reason, would be the god of the role culture or bureaucracy. Handy also makes the point that role cultures are effective as long as the environment within which they operate is stable. In environments which are not controlled and which are changing, bureaucracies, because of their rules, fixed role positions and authority structures are slow to change. In an environment where there is pressure for change, for example in maternity services, it can be seen that achieving that change within current health service bureaucracies will have inherent difficulties.

The task culture is described as a net which is formed and altered to meet the needs of the job. Different people are brought into this type of organisation depending on the job which has to be achieved. Handy describes this type of organisation as being very flexible and responsive to change but difficult to control and is unable to identify a suitable ruling deity for the task culture. The task organisation, or team culture, is in marked contrast to the bureaucratic culture. The final form of organisational culture that Handy describes is the person culture in which the group exists to help the individuals within it. This form is found in architects' partnerships, consultancy firms and other small organisations. The organisation is described as a galaxy of individual stars who have Dionysus as their god: 'the god of the self-orientated individual, the first existentialist' (Handy, 1976, p. 184). In midwifery perhaps some of the group practices of independent midwives or some team midwifery groups could be described as operating within a person culture.

If the different organisations which provide maternity services are considered, features of one or other of these models or a combination of these models may be identified. It can be seen that the structures of maternity services are not unique and that use of these models may help in the identification of common features and characteristics shared by maternity services and other organisations. This knowledge can then help in any movement to make changes in the structures. It can be suggested, for example, that the team approach to maternity care is seeking to move the organisation of maternity services from the bureaucratic, role culture, to the task culture or even the person culture described by Handy (1976).

THE ACTION APPROACH TO ORGANISATIONS

The descriptions above were focused on internal relationships within organisations but, as Handy (1976) acknowledges in relation to the role culture organisation, organisations do not exist in isolation but are part of society and affected by society. Davies and Francis (1976) argue that the professional organisation and bureaucracy models are inadequate to describe the hospital as an organisation and Davies (1979) suggests that organisational theory should consider the interrelationship of health care with other organisations and aspects of society. Silverman (1970) is similarly critical of organisation theory which separates the organisation as a unit from the wider society and considers that a better understanding of organisations may be achieved if the relationships between the organisation and the wider society are specified. Silverman's (1970) action approach to organisations rests on the view that society and thus organisations are socially constructed and dependent on the meanings attached to them by members of the society or the organisation.

Berger and Luckmann (1976) describe this as the social construction of reality, a model which describes the theory developed by symbolic interactionists. Each individual experiences reality differently and constructs their own understanding of reality, or their environment, differently:

> Linking human behaviour with the state of the world in which it exists made it possible to ask how the environment affects its creators and led to the realization that this effect depends on how people experience the environment and that how they experience the environment depends on how they construct it. Individuals are ultimately responsible for the impact of the environment because they learn from personally constructed experience. (Agyris and Schön, 1974, p. xi)

Silverman (1970) contrasts the action approach to organisations, which places the organisation within its social context, with the approach of the bureaucratic and systems models, which reify organisations and separate them from the social context. Systems theories describe organisations as biological systems with certain needs and goals which are achieved by taking in inputs and producing endproducts. All parts of the system are seen as being interdependent and little attention is given within these models to the purposes of individuals within organisations. The professional organisation model, in contrast, concentrates on the relationship between individuals and the power held by different professions. Silverman (1970) argues that neither of these approaches is satisfactory as one emphasises the formal role structure and role position of members of an organisation and ignores their individual values, and the second exaggerates the extent to which individuals seek to achieve their own ends and extend their own power while ignoring the existence of shared values and interdependence (Silverman, 1970).

The model that Silverman (1970) describes as a framework to assist in the analysis and understanding of organisations has four elements: the changing stock of knowledge outside the organisation, in the wider society; the internal organisational role system; the individual's

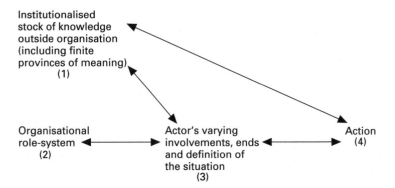

Figure 3.1   *The action approach to organisations*

(Fig 7.1, p. 151, Silverman, 1970. Reproduced with permission of Heinemann
Educational Books Ltd and D. Silverman)

definition of the situation: values, attitudes, attachments, meanings and
the way that the individual understands (constructs) reality which will
be a consequence of their wider experiences and experiences in the organisation; and the actions of individuals which result from the interaction of the other elements as shown in Figure 3.1.

This diagram helps to show that midwifery care, the action, results
from the interaction of a number of factors. Some of the factors which
are relevant to the care of the childbearing woman are illustrated in
Figure 3.2. The values and attitudes in the wider society towards birth,
motherhood, women, families, midwives, the medical profession and
other factors will have an influence on the organisation of maternity
services. The structures within the organisation – for example, the relationships between the different professional groups involved in the care
of the childbearing woman: midwives, obstetricians, physiotherapists
and others, and the management systems, whether these are hierarchical
or collegial – will also affect the activities of midwives and the care of
women.

The knowledge, skills and models of midwifery care held by the
midwives and the women for whom they are caring will also have a
significant influence on the type of care that midwives are able to
provide. For example, if a midwife lacks communication skills, it may
be more difficult for a woman to become an active participant in her
care. If a woman expects health-care professionals to take responsibility for her care, she may react with hostility when asked to assume this
responsibility herself.

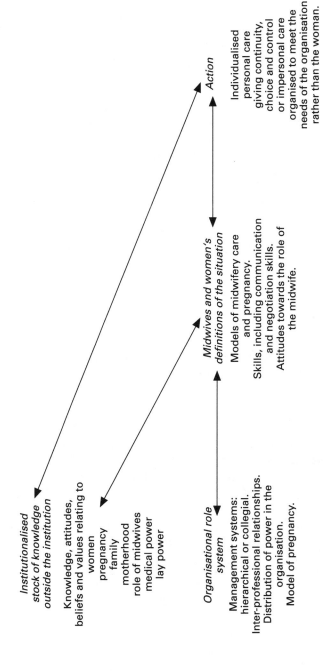

Figure 3.2 *The action framework and care of the childbearing woman*

This conceptual model brings together the different models held by the different parties involved in the provision of midwifery care: the wider society, the hospital/community unit, the individual practitioners, women and their families and suggests ways in which these models may interrelate to produce the action, the care of the childbearing woman. A few examples of different models may help to illustrate this process.

In her study of working-class women, Roberts (1984) interviewed women about their life experiences, including their experiences of childbearing between 1890 and 1940. The social attitudes towards pregnancy and childbirth were influenced by the mortality associated with childbirth and by sexual prudery:

> For many women who had children, pregnancy and confinement were and continued to be a source of both physical and psychological pain throughout the period. Some women (and men) regarded pregnancy as an embarrassment or unclean state. This was yet another aspect of the all-prevailing prudery about sexual matters. (Roberts, 1984, p. 104)

Today mortality has decreased significantly and sexual attitudes have changed greatly in society, changes which have both had a marked effect on the attitudes in the wider society regarding childbirth.

In relation to the models held by individuals Odent (1984) provides an illustration of one model which may be held by some midwives (in particular, those occupying the 'high hard ground' discussed in Chapter 2) and, as he suggests, has a significant impact on the type of care they give:

> Then there are the others, possibly more of them, who unconsciously protect themselves from over-involvement and will offer more impersonal, technical, brisk, mechanical and ultimately 'inhuman' care. They are a bad model for the mother to emulate. The behaviour of some professional staff who have grown too accustomed to the newborn can only be compared with the loveless maternal rearing now known to induce future schizophrenia. (Odent, 1984, p. 90)

Arms (1981) illustrates the effect that the organisational structures may have on care even when the nurse-midwives and other health practitioners hold woman-centred models of care:

> Despite the personal beliefs and intentions of the residents and midwives alike, both are caught in a system that moves women through birth too quickly to permit closeness with any patient.

If nurse-midwives are ever to function as true midwives, they must be free from the pressure to rush and alter the natural process. The average hospital is not conducive to normal birth experiences, even with the finest nurse-midwives and the finest intentions. (Arms, 1981, p. 323)

These illustrations show the effects that the model held about childbirth at societal level, the models held by midwives and the model structuring the organisation may have on the type of care provided to childbearing women. These illustrations also indicate that changes in models are required at different levels if the care women experience is to change. Change at one point cannot be relied on to produce change in care.

Change in care cannot, for example, be produced simply through a change in the knowledge of the midwives within an organisation. In one study which sought to introduce individualised care, efforts were concentrated on increasing midwives' knowledge of individual care and in changing some of their working practices through the allocation of women to each midwife (Adams *et al.*, 1981; Bryar, 1985; 1991a). The evaluation of this study showed that most of the midwives held models of childbearing (their theories-in-action, Agyris and Schön (1974)) that supported the idea of individualised care but, in practice, the type of care that was given was focused on physical needs and on routine needs rather than the individual needs of women (their theories-in-use, Agyris and Schön (1974)). The system within which these midwives worked limited the extent to which they could provide individualised care and actually discouraged individualised care, through the operation of policies and routines that were supported by the structures of the organisation, the professional power relationships and management hierarchies. Change was not attempted in other parts of the organisation, which limited the care which the midwives could provide. The following description shows this process of limiting individualised care in action in the case of a woman who was experiencing a normal labour and who did not wish to be monitored, but who was monitored when the midwife had failed to negotiate successfully with the doctors on behalf of the woman:

In the following example, from the Labour ward, negotiation took place between staff over several hours to meet the individual wishes of the woman which conflicted with the organisational policy that every woman should be monitored when admitted in labour, electronically:

SM X: Do you want her to have a CTG? [cardiotocographic record]

Sr E: No, she does not really want to have one.

11.07 a.m. Dr E (locum) into the room discussing Mrs W with SM X

Dr E: Will you do a CTG?

SM X: She does not really want to have a CTG if it is not necessary.

Dr E replied that having a CTG was not really intervention and went to admit Mrs W. Mrs W managing contractions by relaxation and changing position.

12.30 p.m. Dr E into the room again asking SM X to do a CTG and saying again that it was not intervention. SM X replying that Mrs W did not want anything. Dr E over to Mrs W and telling her that she should have a CTG done and that it was not intervention.

Mrs W: How long for?

Dr E: About 1 hour.

Mrs W: Can I sit up to do it as I would like to sit in the chair?

Dr E: It is better in bed. (Continued discussing reasons for the CTG)

Mrs W: If I want to can I get up? (Getting up on hands and knees)

Dr E leaving room.

12.37 p.m. SM X to office to write up Obstetric Notes prior to the handover report.

Dr F (senior registrar) into office, reading Mrs W's Notes, saying to SM X: Do I understand she is anti-monitoring?

SM X: She just does not want any intervention that is not necessary. She wants to manage on her own, walking about.

Dr F: I'd like her to have a CTG.

SM X: I'll do it for 20 minutes then.

Dr F: Yes, as long as it's done.

12.42 p.m. SM X back to Mrs W and telling her that she will put the CTG on for 20 minutes. Mrs W asking if she could sit in the chair.

SM X: Will sit you up in bed.

13.00 putting on CTG bands. Mrs W complaining that they were too tight, loosened several times. SM X showing Mr W the heartbeat and the contractions on the trace. (Observation Notes, Labour Ward). (Bryar, 1985, pp. 292–3)

This example illustrates many different facets of care but in its very or-dinariness it shows the effect of the medical model, expressed in the concern of the doctors that a policy should be fulfilled though there was no evidence that this woman particularly needed to be monitored.

Currently in Britain there is great pressure at the level of society to achieve change in services for childbearing women (House of

Commons Health Committee, 1992; Department of Health, 1993a and 1993b). A dramatic change can be seen to be taking place in the model held at society level which is seeking to achieve change in the organisations and individuals providing midwifery and obstetric care, as well as in those receiving such care. The action approach to organisations demonstrates the need to attend to the constraints on change at the level of society, the organisation (and all the groups within the organisation) and the individual. For example, what consequences do the following 'Indicators of Success' (actions) have for these three points in the model?

1. All women should be entitled to carry their own notes.
6. Midwives should have direct access to some beds in all maternity units. (Department of Health, 1993a, p. 70)

Depending on the models held by the midwives, obstetricians, health service managers, women and their families, these indicators or actions will be more or less difficult to attain in different places.

Throughout the remainder of this book the concern is with the consequences of different models for practice, for the action of midwives. The action approach to organisations is used throughout the book as the model underpinning this discussion of the action, the care by midwives. The model helps to clarify why it is important that midwives are able to articulate their models of practice. If these models can be articulated they can then be examined in relation to the prevailing models in society and the models held by other occupational groups and the women and their families. Difficulties in achieving the aims of midwifery care may then be more easily identified along with ways of seeking to achieve change.

MODELS AND CHANGE

It may be argued that the introduction or adoption of a model for midwifery practice involves little change, evolution rather than revolution, and in some situations this may be the case, as Roach and Brown (1991) describe. Consideration of the action approach to organisations indicates, however, that if the philosophy of an organisation is going to be changed, if the model on which it operates is going to change, this will have fundamental effects on all aspects of the organisation. If the model envisaged in recent government reports is to become a reality, changes will be required in the organisational role system if midwives are to actually work as independent practitioners. Changes will be needed in education if new students and those already practising are going to be able to take on new responsibilities, and changes will also be required in the preparation of doctors and other health professionals. Changes will be needed in systems of antenatal, intranatal and postnatal care and women and their families will have to be involved in the decisions about these changes. The introduction of a different model requires fundamental change, change which may not be welcomed by all (Chapman, 1985).

Marris (1986) describes three types of change: sudden and unexpected; revolutionary; and planned change. Changes in organisations in which midwifery care is provided should not be sudden and unexpected (although without careful planning this is how many may view change). The change is rarely revolutionary, in the sense Marris (1986) uses it, involving violence and destruction, but it may be revolutionary in the sense that the change in philosophy demonstrates a huge change in thinking. Rather, change in health care organisations is generally planned. Hegyvary (1982) describes planned change as follows: 'It starts with the first presentation of an idea to a group, and, if successful, it ends when the new idea is integrated into the culture of the group' (p. 12).

Planned change may be achieved through the use of one of three approaches or a combination of the three (Chin and Benne, 1976, cited by Hegyvary, 1982). The empirical-rational approach to change suggests that if people are presented with information they will change their behaviour if they see the new behaviour as being beneficial. The normative-reeducative approach suggests that, although the presentation of information is important, people will not make changes unless their attitudes and values are changed. The third approach to change, the power-coercive, depends on the exercise of power on those with less power forcing them to make changes. In considering changes in models of practice held by midwives it has to be remembered that the model that the individual holds is very personal to them. Changes in the model held by an individual will therefore require changes in values and attitudes which may best be achieved through the normative-reeducative approach. Change at the organisational level, where fundamental organisational change is sought, also requires changes in hearts and minds, in values and attitudes, again more likely to be achieved through normative-reeducative change.

Lewin (1952) concentrates on the achievement of normative-reeducative change and is concerned with the effects of group membership on change. In a study of the use of cod-liver oil and orange juice by new mothers Lewin found that women who received advice about these supplements in a group were more likely to give them to their babies than women who received this information in individual consultations. Lewin describes the process of change as change in the individual's attachment to particular rules through a process of unfreezing, moving and refreezing which may be facilitated by group membership:

1. [Education] must alter the cognitive structure, the person's facts, beliefs, expectations, and ways of seeing the physical and social worlds.
2. It must modify values and principles about what the person should or should not do, as well as the person's feelings about status and authority and his attractions and aversions to other groups and their standards.
3. It must introduce new motoric actions, a new repertoire of behavioural skills and conscious control of body movements and social actions. (Hegyvary, 1982, p. 12)

Change thus requires change in beliefs, in the picture or model of care, and change in actions, in the care given. This description identifies the need for people, in this case midwives, to be given the opportunity (if they do not have the skills already) to develop new skills, for example, in adult education or methods of helping women to participate in their care. This model of change also suggests that change within organisations may be a very slow process, as it is dependent on internalisation of the model, or change, by each individual and each individual coming to terms with the change.

Marris (1986) considers that the change process requires careful management if long-term problems are to be avoided both by the individual and the organisation, and if real change is to be achieved. Marris (1986) undertook studies of change involved in bereavement, rehousing and other situations and considers that in all these situations individuals seek to maintain continuity in their environments and their lives. The way we behave is dependent on our past experiences through which we have developed our beliefs and attitudes. Change threatens to break this continuity and people will make attempts to maintain or restore continuity, to restore the meanings that have underpinned their lives.

Change is described by Marris (1986) in terms of the degree to which it disrupts the individual's understanding of the world and the balance between continuity, growth and loss in relation to past experiences. The first type of change is substitutional and does not disrupt the meanings of life. The second type represents growth but the changes can still be incorporated into the current meanings of life. The third type of change is potentially destructive, entailing loss and discontinuity. Obviously the same change may be viewed in different ways by different individuals. For example, the midwife who has always sought to provide individualised care will welcome the chance to work as a member of a small team with a caseload, whereas the midwife who has been meticulous about the detailed organisation of the structures of the antenatal clinic may find it less easy to accept the less structured way of working implicit in working in a midwifery team which has the aim of providing women with individualised care. Individuals build up expectations and patterns of behaviour, of how they view themselves as midwives and how they view childbirth and care of the childbearing woman, and any change, whether welcomed or not, will disrupt this understanding:

> Change threatens to invalidate this experience, robbing them of the skills they have learned and confusing their purposes, upsetting the subtle rationalisations and compensations by which they reconciled the different aspects of their situation. (Marris, 1986, p. 157)

Marris (1986) suggests that much change can be understood as a process of bereavement, in which taken-for-granted meanings are disrupted. Like the bereaved person, the person involved in change needs time to work through their feelings about the change. They need to have the opportunity to express anger or despair, to question and challenge the change and work through the process of loss involved in any change, however welcome that change. In studies of the introduction of the nursing process and primary nursing Mead and Bryar (1992) identified reactions of fear and personal threat; denial; pinning; bargaining; loss of predictability; and loss of self resulting from the changes. The person involved in introducing change, for example introducing a new model of care, needs to understand this process of reaction and adoption or rejection of change. Many change agents take personal responsibility for the failure of change to take place but Marris (1986) helps to demonstrate the commonalities in all changes that are outside the control of the change agent but which must be attended to by the change agent to prevent harm to those being encouraged to change, or failure of the change.

New models of care require changes in thinking, in values and beliefs, in organisational structures, in societal attitudes and in actions, in practice. Such changes need to be handled with awareness and care.

THE ORGANISATION OF MATERNITY SERVICES IN THE NETHERLANDS AND MIDWIFERY CARE

In the first part of this chapter a model, the action approach to organisations, was discussed which identifies the interrelationships of the models of care held by different parts of the organisation on the care experienced by the childbearing woman. In this section the type of care provided in the Netherlands is discussed as an illustration of the effect that a different model of childbearing in society has on maternity services.

The following description perhaps lays emphasis on the differences between the maternity services in the Netherlands and Britain but it needs to be remembered that the services in the Netherlands are not uniform. There are high-tech hospitals as well as highly-developed homebirth services provided, in general, by self-employed midwives although in some areas provided through midwives employed by local authorities. As in Britain, the needs of society for low-cost services (an influence at the societal level) provides constant pressure on midwifery care. Competition between the large number of general practitioners and obstetricians (who are also independent contractors) and midwives for care of women also affects the care that midwives are able to provide (Benoit, 1992).

The philosophy underpinning the maternity services in the Netherlands is that pregnancy and childbirth are natural, physiological processes. As Kloosterman (1984) comments: 'The system is based on the belief that human parturition belongs in principle to such activities as breathing and laughing' (p. 115). This social attitude has resulted in a system which supports homebirth, the role of the midwife as a practitioner in normal birth and the ability of women to give birth and to be in control of the birth process. This approach to the organisation of maternity services produces the following characteristics (actions): over 33 per cent of births take place at home; midwives work in independent practice and a low-technology approach is evident in the practice of the midwives, general practitioners and the obstetricians (Smulders and Limburg, 1988).

There are six factors which underpin the organisation of the maternity services and which can be located in relation to the action approach to organisations:

(1) the cultural environment in the Netherlands which views birth as a normal process which should take place at home (institutionalised stock of knowledge);

(2) the legal position of the midwife as an independent practitioner whose practice is proscribed by law (an additional indicator of the social attitude towards midwives) (institutionalised stock of knowledge and the organisational role system);
(3) the national antenatal screening system (organisational role system);
(4) the assistance provided during homebirths to the midwife and the care provided postnatally to the childbearing woman and her family by maternity home care assistants (institutionalised role system and actors' definitions of the situation);
(5) the insurance system (institutionalised stock of knowledge and the organisational role system);
(6) that community midwives, general practitioners and obstetricians are entrepreneurs in independent practice (Bryar, 1991b; Teijlingen van, 1991) (organisational role system and actors' definitions of the system).

Smulders and Limburg (1988) describe the historical development of midwifery in the Netherlands and the attitude of cooperation rather than competition which existed between midwives, general practitioners and academic doctors (who later became obstetricians) in the nineteenth century. This degree of cooperation was in marked contrast to the suppression and hostility experienced by midwives in other countries (Donnison, 1988; Sullivan and Weitz, 1988). In 1865 a law was passed in the Netherlands which defined the area of practice of midwives and doctors involved in maternity care.

Midwives were made the lead professionals in the care of women experiencing normal deliveries and had status as practitioners of normal midwifery. Smulders and Limburg (1988) contrast the position of the midwife with that of the nurse, commenting that:

> A nurse has to work within the hierarchy of the hospital, under the supervision of doctors. A midwife on the other hand, has equivalent rights in the field of obstetrics as general practitioners and she is expected to work independently in the field. (Smulders and Limburg, 1988, p. 239)

The law provided the context for that independent practice through a payment system which limited payment for care of the woman with a normal pregnancy to midwives. The state also regulated the education of midwives through the establishment of three schools for midwifery education (the first opened in 1861). Education for midwives is currently provided in three centres and lasts three years (Teijlingen van and McCaffery, 1987). The state, society, therefore determined the extent of practice of midwives and established education to enable midwives to provide the type of care that society required for women experiencing a normal pregnancy.

This legislation restricted the involvement of doctors in the care of women with a normal pregnancy through preventing them from gaining payment for this care. By doing this the legislation limited the power of the medical profession over midwives and women. As they were not paid for care of women with a normal pregnancy, doctors were less interested in their care and were inhibited in extending their practice to care of these women, although sections of the medical profession in the Netherlands have sought, from time to time, to extend their practice to care for this group of women. In Britain and other countries medical practice was not controlled in this way and expanded into care of the woman with an uncomplicated pregnancy, reducing the area of practice of the midwife. Many British midwives would, probably, recognise their own position in the description of the position of the nurse described by Smulders and Limburg (1988) above. Through legislation, an act by society reflecting the attitudes and knowledge in society, the organisational role system in the Netherlands has been affected and the professional dominance of one professional group over another has been limited.

The care of women in pregnancy is determined by antenatal screening. The screening process selects women who should have a hospital birth (Teijlingen van, 1992). This contrasts with the approach to maternity care in Britain, which is based on the assumption that all women will give birth in a hospital and where homebirth may be viewed as 'anti-social behaviour by a self-neglecting subculture' (Offerman, 1985, cited by Kitzinger, 1988, p. 231). The system of antenatal screening was developed by Professor Kloosterman and others and is regularly updated (Teijlingen van, 1992). Using a combination of physiological and social measures, women are screened to determine if they are at high risk of developing complications, in which case they are referred for care by an obstetrician. Midwives are not allowed to care for women at high risk. Women who are expected to have a normal pregnancy may be cared for by a midwife or a general practitioner. Women attend for an average of 12 antenatal visits and can be transferred to care of the obstetrician at any time during pregnancy.

Following birth, women are cared for at home for up to eight days both by their midwife and Maternity Home Care Assistants who assist at homebirths and in all aspects of care of the home and family postnatally (Teijlingen van, 1992). The maternity assistants provide practical support, advice and health education enabling the midwife (who has a considerable caseload, as discussed below) to concentrate on other aspects of care as Oppenheimer (1993) comments: 'The midwife visits for consultation only' (p. 1401). Van Teijlingen (1990) states: 'Dutch midwives and GPs are glad that they can leave most of the nursing and caring tasks to the Maternity Home Care Assistants' (p. 361). Smulders and Limburg (1988) describe the Maternity Home Care Assistants keeping notes of events in the postnatal period which are then discussed with the midwife and parents on the midwife's visits.

The provision of Maternity Home Care Assistants since 1925 (Smulders and Limburg, 1988) indicates the value placed by society on care of women after delivery and appreciation of their need for support both with caring for themselves and their family and learning about their baby. This provision also acknowledges that midwives cannot spend a great deal of time with each woman on postnatal visits. In Britain the tradition has been for midwives to undertake most of the postnatal care although, in some parts of the country, home helps used to be available to help women in the early postnatal period. Towler and Bramall (1986) and Leap and Hunter (1993) describe the extensive 'nursing' care that midwives provided up to the 1960s for women who remained on enforced bed-rest postnatally for many days. This extensive postnatal care contrasts with the limited antenatal care that was provided early in the twentieth century to women in Britain. In the Netherlands the focus on detailed antenatal care may have contributed to the subsequent development of a midwifery auxiliary (or health care assistant) to undertake home postnatal care. Van Teijlingen (1992) notes that midwives in the Netherlands each care for 100–250 women per annum (assisting at the births of, on average, 160 of these women) and comments that: 'The Dutch maternity services could not have survived without their [the Maternity Home Care Assistants'] existence' (p. 3). As changes are made in the organisation of maternity services in Britain and in the work of midwives, the work of the Maternity Home Care Assistants needs to be considered carefully within the context of the overall organisation of maternity services.

Health care in the Netherlands is funded through a variety of insurance systems (Ministry of Welfare, Health and Cultural Affairs, 1987). Since the act of 1865 midwives' income for homebirths has been protected and they are paid from the Sick Funds (Teijlingen van and McCaffery, 1987). Midwives are the only health professionals who are paid for care of a woman experiencing a normal pregnancy. A general practitioner only receives payment for such care if there is no midwife working in the area, and obstetricians do not get paid for such care but only get paid for caring for women with a high-risk pregnancy (Teijlingen van, 1991). This means that the income of midwives is protected but it also limits the choice of women as to which health professional will provide care. Smulders and Limburg (1988, p. 239) comment that this system of payment has been under attack for many years, from the medical profession, but it has continued because the government (society) wants to preserve the 'institution of midwifery' (p. 239). It may also have continued due to the differential costs associated with care by midwives and care by doctors. In Britain the income of an obstetrician from the NHS is £50 000 while the average income of a midwife is £15 000 (Pallot, 1993).

Midwives, general practitioners and obstetricians in the Netherlands are all independent contractors, entrepreneurs or small businesses in the same way as general practitioners are in Britain. As such they are all in competition with each other although the legal restrictions on the role of the midwife and the payments system, described above, limit this competition to some extent. The legal protection of the role of the midwife provides protection, status and income but also limits practice as Van Teijlingen and McCaffery (1987) describe, to the normal with referral, and relinquishing of care, if any abnormality is detected. Competition between midwives and obstetricians may inhibit midwives from making referrals to obstetricians who are seen to retain the care of women once they have been referred, both for medical reasons and possibly for financial reasons in that they, rather than the midwife will receive the payment for the care (Teijlingen van and McCaffery, 1987).

Doctors may use various arguments to retain the care of a woman once she has been referred, reinforcing her concerns about her pregnancy (Teijlingen van and McCaffery, 1987) and reducing her confidence in herself. McKay (1993) describes Astrid Limburg's description of this process: 'Limburg characterizes the doctor's attitude as "trust me" – that is, for the woman to look to the doctor rather than her own ability to give birth, and women consequently lose their confidence' (p. 119). Smulders and Limburg (1988) make the point, however, that the position of midwives in the Netherlands has been assisted at crucial times by the support of influential obstetricians. This type of support is demonstrated, for example, in the writings of Professor Kloosterman (1984) in his support for homebirths and the view that the midwife's role is to assist in the normal process of childbirth.

Another means to restrict competition between entrepreneurs is to limit entry into the occupational group. This has been done in the Netherlands where there were only 949 midwives in 1986, 695 practising independently, serving a population of approximately 14.9 million (Smulders and Limburg, 1988). There are therefore 63 midwives for every one million of the population in the Netherlands, compared to 2159 midwives to every one million of the population in Britain (Teijlingen van, 1993). This figure is based on the estimate by Flint (1993, pp. 59–60) that there are 22 666 midwives in clinical practice in England and Wales and the 1991 preliminary census count of a population of 48 925 000 in England and Wales (Teijlingen van, 1993). Flint (1993) estimates that 19 740 midwives in England and Wales, with caseloads of 36 women per annum, would be able to provide continuity of care to all childbearing women with the remainder of midwives providing a skeleton staff in hospital and providing intensive care to those who need such care. Ball *et al.* (1992) provide additional information on the structural conditions that would be needed for more independent midwifery practice.

McKay (1993) suggests that further pressures are being placed on midwives in the Netherlands by the growth in the numbers of obstetric specialists and the extent to which Dutch midwives are overworked and underpaid in relation to the payments that are made to specialists. She comments that additional pressures may be placed on midwives by the introduction of a market economy into health care in which the position of the midwife as the lead professional in care of women with a normal pregnancy would no longer be protected.

This example demonstrates the importance of the social context of health care. For nearly 130 years the special place of the midwife in Dutch society has been protected by the payment system. This era could be ended by the introduction of competition and a market economy. The extent to which midwives would survive in a market economy would then be dependent on the attitudes of the users of the services and the extent to which other models of pregnancy, for example the medical model, managed to gain ground in a society which has viewed pregnancy and childbirth largely as a natural process (see Chapter 5). The issue of the introduction of a free market is of interest in the current debate in Britain about the structure of maternity services. The purchaser–provider divide has the potential to give new opportunities for midwives to establish independent practices and to negotiate contracts with health purchasers to provide maternity services. However, evidence from the Netherlands suggests that a free market approach to the provision of midwifery care may result in less personal care and burnt-out midwives who might have to take on large caseloads to achieve a reasonable salary unless there is some way of providing them with a protected salary (Benoit, 1992).

The social system in the Netherlands has supported and maintained the position of the midwife through a philosophy of care that supports the view of pregnancy as a normal life event (Oppenheimer, 1993). Legislation has limited the area of practice of medicine, a powerful professional group competing with midwives for care of childbearing women. The organisational role system has provided a legally defined area of practice for midwives who have status and responsibilities equivalent to general practitioners, and restriction of entrants into the profession of midwifery has limited their number. Professional support from other role occupants, such as leading obstetricians, has contributed to midwives maintaining their role, as has the work of the Maternity Home Care Assistants. Independent practice in singlehanded or small group practices has enabled midwives to exercise their philosophy of care; as Smulders and Limburg (1988) put it, the childbearing woman is a healthy person who, with assistance, 'will achieve something very special' (p. 241). And the attitude among women and their families has been that childbirth is a normal process, as the following comment from a Dutch woman illustrates: 'I discussed it with many people, who invariably all had sisters or grandchildren who had all been delivered without any problems. I never heard one negative story. Some people said: "I was born that way and I look well, don't I?"' (Rees van, *et al.*, 1984)

The system of care in the Netherlands is very different from that in Britain but recent government reports (House of Commons Health Committee, 1992; Department of Health, 1993a) suggest that maternity services should adopt a model in some ways similar to that in the Netherlands. The discussion has highlighted the complex interrelationship of the total system of maternity care and the need to attend to the many different aspects of the organisation when change is being instituted. In this discussion the use of the action approach to organisations can be seen to limit the areas considered. According to Handy (1976), consideration of change could require attention to 60 or more aspects affecting organisations which may require attention if change in maternity care (the action) is to be achieved. The discussion also highlights the dynamic nature of organisations, that organisations are constantly changing. A number of threats to the present system of care in the Netherlands has been identified, showing that changes in one area, for example the attitude of society to midwives or rising health care costs, can have a profound effect on other aspects of the organisation and the care provided. Kloosterman (1984) summarises the difficulties in providing protection to the two groups of childbearing women, the need for an integrated approach by all those in the maternity services to achieve this care, and the difficulties of developing such a system:

(1) Protection of a small minority of all mothers and children against the dangers of pregnancy and childbirth by all the achievements of modern medicine.

(2) Protection of the great majority of all mothers and children against human meddlesomeness and endeavours to change a normal physiological act into an operation.

> To achieve this, we need a strong organisation for midwifery supported by the Government, the medical establishment and, last but not least, the expectant mothers themselves. It is difficult enough to keep such an organisation intact when it already exists, let alone to start one *de novo*. (Kloosterman, 1984, p. 125)

Summary

The aim of this chapter has been to describe the influence of different factors on midwifery care. The organisational context of midwifery care has been described and the action framework, or model, suggested as one means of understanding the different factors affecting the action, care of the childbearing woman. Midwifery care occurs within a complex social situation and any changes in that care must take into account the other factors influencing midwifery practice, apart from the attributes of individual midwives. The process of change has been described as a process similar to the process of grief. When change is introduced there is a need for each individual to reintegrate the change into their understanding of the world. Finally the organisation of the maternity services in the Netherlands was described. The maternity services in the Netherlands are provided within a society in which the model of pregnancy as a normal life event is prevalent. This has effects on the organisation of the maternity services at government level in the payment system, in the expectations of women of their care and in the practice of midwives in independent practices.

Activities

Using the material in this chapter as a basis, consider the following questions in relation to your own practice.

1 In your everyday practice, whose needs predominate in the type of care you are able to provide?

2 What are the effects of the hospital, team, community or other setting in which you practice on the care you are able to provide?

3 Would you describe yourself as a pre-professional, technocrat or professional (using Benoit's (1987) terms)?

4 With reference to the types of organisation described by Handy (1976) what type of organisation do you work within?

5 With reference to the action framework, identify the main factors which influence the type of care you are able to provide.

6 Describe an example of individualised care and identify the factors which supported or inhibited this care.

7 '1. All women should be entitled to carry their own notes.
6. Midwives should have direct access to some beds in all maternity units. (Department of Health, 1993a).'
Consider these aims and, using the action framework, describe any changes that would be needed to achieve these aims.

8 Think of a time in which you have been involved in change. How was that change presented to you and what were your reactions to that change? How would you manage the change process in the future?

9 How does the system of maternity care in the Netherlands provide continuity, choice and control for women?

10 What features of the maternity services in the Netherlands, if any, do you consider should be incorporated into the maternity services in Britain and how could this be achieved?

11 Describe the model of pregnancy which underpins the organisation within which you work.

CHAPTER FOUR

Models and theories influencing midwifery care

In all his writings, Grantley Dick-Read spoke not of a 'method' of childbirth, but of a philosophy of life, of which birth is just a part, although a most essential part. He believed that the quality of the birth experience influenced (for good or ill) not only the child, but the family into which he or she was born. He stated that the childbirth practices of a nation were reflections of that nation's beliefs concerning the integrity and dignity of life, and influenced that nation for good or ill, and that ultimately the world itself is affected. (Wessel and Ellis, 1987, p. 2)

INTRODUCTION

In this chapter, two models, a theory and a concept which influence or underpin midwifery practice and which have been developed in other areas of practice or other disciplines, will be considered. As discussed in Chapter 3, the actions of midwives, midwifery care, result from the interaction of the models of childbirth and midwifery held within society, in the health care organisation and by the individual midwife. It is therefore important to consider those models, theories and concepts which have an impact on the environment within which midwifery is practised and which will have an effect on that practice.

The range of disciplines, theories and models on which midwifery practice draws, and which influence the environment of care of the childbearing woman, is enormous as examination of midwifery and other texts shows. The following provide some examples:

Sociology: role theory (Jenson *et al.*, 1977); symbolic interaction theory (Moore, 1983); exchange theory (Moore, 1983); systems theory (Moore, 1983); conflict theory (Moore, 1983); functionalism (Moore, 1983); change theory (Auvenshine and Enriquez, 1990); a sociology of childbirth (Oakley, 1980).

Physiology: of pregnancy, labour and the puerperium (Bennett and Brown, 1993; Silverton, 1993).

Anthropology: cross-cultural theories (Moore, 1983); culture shock (Moore, 1983); culture change (Moore, 1983); rites of passage (Littlewood, 1989).

Psychology: theories relating to all aspects of childbearing and the newborn baby (Prince and Adams, 1987); models of helping and coping (Cronewett and Brickman (1982); postnatal depression (Oakley and Chamberlain, 1981; Beck, 1993).

Health promotion: theory and methods of health promotion (Murphy-Black and Faulkner, 1988; Combes and Schonveld, 1992; Ewles and Simnett, 1992; Dines and Cribb, 1993).

Adult education: theory and practice relating to learning and teaching (Kolb, 1984; Boud *et al.*, 1985; Combes and Schonveld, 1992; O'Meara, 1993).

Feminism: feminist influences in midwifery (Kirkham, 1986; McCool and McCool, 1989).

History of midwifery: origins, development and future of midwifery (Walker, 1976; Towler and Bramall, 1986; Donnison, 1988).

Teamwork: the theory and reality of teamwork (Belbin, 1981; Adair, 1986; Bennett and Brown, 1993; Flint, 1993; Wraight *et al.*, 1993).

The above lists and subject areas are by no means exhaustive but provide an idea of the vast range of knowledge and theory which informs and enriches the environment within which midwifery care is provided. A number of these models and theories have been referred to in earlier chapters but it would clearly be impossible to examine each and the consequences of each for midwifery care here. Instead, a number have been selected for discussion which operate at one or more points in the action framework discussed in Chapter 3.

The medical model is an example of a model which is extremely influential at the level of information in society, as well as having a significant impact on the structure of organisations, and the individual perceptions of people using those organisations, for example during pregnancy, and those working in health care organisations, for example midwives. Bonding theory may be stated most baldly in the form: *if* the mother and baby are together during the sensitive period after birth *then* bonding will take place. The contrary statement of this theory (that if the mother and baby are not together) has had a significant impact on the organisation of maternity services. Bonding theory is considered as an example of theory which had a significant impact on the organisation and humanisation of maternity services.

The Health for All model, another model operating at the level of society, has a pervasive and increasing, although possibly less well-recognised effect on the present and future organisation of maternity services. Finally, one concept, participation, which forms part of the model of Health for All is discussed with a view to defining the meanings given to this concept. Participation is a facet of care generally considered to be mainly affected by the actions and beliefs of the individual (the individual's definition of the situation) but which is either supported or undermined by the structure of the organisation and attitudes in society. The need for the definition of concepts was considered in Chapter 2 as a precursor for measurement of the extent to which the concept is evident in practice. Participation is one element, or concept, in the model of midwifery care which seeks to achieve continuity, choice and control. To achieve participation and to measure whether participation (choice and control) are occurring requires an understanding and definition of this multi-faceted concept.

THE MEDICAL MODEL

The medical model is of great importance to midwifery care, as the influence of this model pervades society, health care organisations and the educational preparation of many health care practitioners. When alternative models of practice are being discussed it is necessary to have a thorough understanding of this important model.

> A practising physician is an actor, not a scholar or philosopher. He needs a conceptual model but one that reduces the reality with which he deals to the bare essentials. If this model is useful in the sense of providing him with serviceable tools, he does not care too much about its oversimplicity and poor correspondence with the external reality. The medical model has served him admirably in this respect. (Vouri and Rimpela, 1981, p. 227)

The medical model is the fundamental model underpinning much midwifery practice. This statement may not be acceptable to many midwives and, indeed, may be offensive to some. However, many midwives would agree that the influence of the medical model is so pervasive in society and in health care organisations that it has to be recognised, faced and addressed before any discussion can be held about other models of midwifery practice and ways of introducing other models into the organisations in which midwifery care occurs.

The purpose of a model is to provide a framework for understanding and action. Two questions can be asked about any model: can it be understood relatively easily and can it be used in practice? Vouri and Rimpela (1981) argue that the medical model meets both these criteria, and its success and world-wide use are the result of its utility in helping doctors to understand human beings, the disease process and ways of intervening to limit the effects of diseases. The medical model provides doctors with a way of understanding the world but, equally, it provides people with a way of understanding medical practice and their relationship to medical practitioners. As McKeown (1989) shows in his description of the new medical student, in Britain and many other parts of the world, members of the population share a particular understanding of medicine which is based on the medical model:

> Their ideas reflect the predominant notions in society about the work of the doctor: that he is concerned with the diagnosis and treatment of disease of individual patients, that most patients are cured by treatment and that it is on medical intervention that health primarily depends. (McKeown, 1989, p. 147)

The medical model is one model which has been developed to help people understand the process of ill-health and the means by which health may be restored. Health and the restoration of health are fundamental to the well-being of communities, and models which help to provide an explanation of illness and health and indicate ways to prevent illness and to help restore people to health if they become unwell are clearly important. There are, as Stacy (1988) describes, other models which provide an understanding of the disease process in other cultures, including the influence of ill-wishing by others, supernatural powers or external events that are identified as the causal agents of the person's ill-health. However, in all cultures, the Western medical model has had great influence and has been utilised worldwide by medical practitioners, many of whom, as Vouri and Rimpela (1981) comment, will have been educated in medical schools in the West.

What then are the main elements of the medical model and what consequences does this model have for practice? Schein (1974), in a study of the education of professionals, identifies three elements which, combined, describe the knowledge base of a profession:

1. An *underlying discipline* or *basic science* component upon which the practice rests or from which it is developed.
2. An *applied science* or *'engineering'* component from which many of the day-to-day diagnostic procedures and problem solutions are derived.

3. A *skills* and *attitudinal* component that concerns actual performance of services to the client, using the underlying basic and
   applied knowledge. (Schein, 1972, p. 43)

These three types of knowledge are demonstrated in the education
and practice of medicine. Underlying theory of, for example, the
disease process, is applied in the diagnosis of the disease by individual
doctors using their interpersonal skills. Schein (1972) argues that, as
professions mature, they become more specialised in their knowledge
base and practice, they become more bureaucratic and more convergent
in the application of knowledge: that is, there is a high degree of agreement about the knowledge base for practice. The knowledge base for
medicine is largely convergent in that there is agreement that the basic
sciences and disciplines such as anatomy, physiology and biochemistry
form key disciplines for medical practice. Schein (1972) contrasts this
position with that of social work, where the knowledge base is more di-
vergent, with different approaches to social work resting on different
branches of psychology, sociology and other disciplines. This analysis
could equally be applied to midwifery, in which there is a similar eclec-
tic use of underlying disciplines and theory.

Medicine is a mature profession which demonstrates a high degree of
specialisation, bureaucratisation and convergence in its knowledge
base. Combining this analysis with the action approach to organisations, it can seen that some of the negative attributes of the medical
model, such as reduction of the person to systems or an impersonal approach by the doctor, may be located in the model and the initial education of the doctor based on this model. These negative attributes and
behaviours may then be reinforced by the organisations within which
medicine is practised, which are structured around the concepts of the
medical model.

Vouri and Rimpela (1981) provide a detailed description of the evolution of the medical model, or discipline, which is comprised of a need
to understand the relationship of human beings with nature, the nature
of the working of the body and the nature of disease. The medical
model has developed over the centuries from the earliest Greek and
Roman practitioners, and one of its strengths is, of course, this long
period of development and gestation. McKeown (1989) discusses
Dubos's (1960) description of the two traditions in medicine which
stem from these early times: those that followed Asclepius
(Aesculapius) whose teaching was that the role of medicine is to treat
disease and to correct imperfections; and those that followed Hygieia
and the teaching that the role of medicine is to understand the natural

laws of health and that 'health is the natural order of things, a positive attribute to which men are entitled if they govern their lives wisely' (McKeown, 1989, p. 3).

Tension has always existed between these two views. The 'medical model', while comprising aspects of both these traditions, is mainly concerned with the tradition of Asclepius, with a focus on the individual and the parts of an individual. Judeo-Christian teachings, in the northern hemisphere, provided the rationale for human beings to see themselves as controlling, rather than controlled by nature, in the belief that human beings had been created in God's image and that it was God's will that human beings use nature for the good of all people (Vouri and Rimpela, 1981). Within this tradition a function of medicine and of sciences in general was therefore to understand and use nature to the benefit of human beings.

The second element in the medical model is the mechanistic view that the model takes of human beings and the way that the human being, the machine, can then be controlled. The philosopher Descartes in the seventeenth century described the body in terms of a machine, although an understanding of the mechanical workings of the body had been developing over many centuries:

> He [Descartes] conceived of the body as a machine, governed almost entirely by the laws of physics, which might be taken apart and re-assembled if its structure and function were understood. (McKeown, 1989, p. 4)

McKeown (1989) comments that discoveries, such as that by Harvey of the mechanical circulation system of blood, reinforced and supported this mechanical model of the body. While this mechanical, take-it-apart, Lego model, has certain attractions in giving direction to research, it has other consequences in the practice of patient care or care of the childbearing woman. It provides a rationale for focusing on one aspect of the individual, for example, the abdomen and the pregnancy, while ignoring other aspects which may be seen as unconnected, for example the woman's dental health or anxieties about the future.

McKeown (1989) considers that another consequence of this model is the conclusion that might, and has been drawn, that any improvements in health of the community are a result of interventions in relation to individuals rather than interventions at the level of society. In *The Role of Medicine*, McKeown (1989) discusses the evidence for the impact of medical care on health and contrasts this with evidence of the improvements in health achieved through improvements in nutrition, sanitation and the control of other environmental factors.

In relation to the health of childbearing women the traditional medical model argument of effectiveness is illustrated by inflexible systems of antenatal care which are based on the proposition that attendance by individual women for ten-plus antenatal examinations will reduce perinatal mortality. The social health model which McKeown (1989) describes attributes improvements in perinatal outcome to improvements in diet, education and other factors as well as medical interventions.

The third element in the medical model is the understanding of the nature of diseases. Stacy (1988) provides a description of the systems of belief about disease causation in Britain in the Middle Ages and the importance of beliefs in good and evil powers, in the power of healing and in the Galenic tradition of the four humours and efforts to restore balance in the humours when someone was ill. Paracelsus, working in the sixteenth century, is identified as the person who changed the focus of attention from the cause of the disease (for example, an outside spiritual influence) to the disease itself, thus helping to change the focus of medical attention from the patient to the disease – the disease process being seen as independent of the patient (Stacy, 1988, p. 38). Scientific discoveries, in particular the discovery and understanding of cell structure, increased knowledge of the process of disease. This understanding continues to grow today with the increasing knowledge, for example, of the effects of genetic factors on disease. Cell theory, that 'the essence of disease was to be found in the altered functioning of cells' (Vuori and Rimpela, 1981, p. 222), had consequences for the practice of medicine and the relationship of the medical practitioner and the person who was unwell:

> This development did, however, help to consign to oblivion the man in whom the disease occurs. When pathological knowledge increased, the holistic concept of man became less necessary as an explanatory variable. Metaphorically, man was forgotten at the dissection table when the scholars focused their attention on the ever more narrowly defined locus of disease. Organs, tissues, and cells could be removed from the body and studied separately, using the unaided eye and later the increasingly sophisticated apparatus. In this endeavour, man was just a mere nuisance in that he could not be put under the microscope. (Vouri and Rimpela, 1981, p. 222)

This compartmentalisation has significant effects on medical practice and on the practice of other health care practitioners who hold this model. The narrow focus is in opposition to holistic care, and the focus on the disease and the part that is diseased has the consequence of helping medicine to be largely reactive rather than proactive and preventive in its practice. The medical practitioner is there to react and treat when something has gone wrong, the 'fire brigade approach' (Macdonald, 1993, p. 34): 'The emphasis is on waiting for something to go wrong; the sufferer then approaches the medical professional, the problem is diagnosed and dealt with' (Macdonald, 1993, p. 34).

The three main elements of the medical model are summarised by Vouri and Rimpela (1981) as the control of nature by human beings; a mechanistic view of human beings; and an understanding of disease which separates human beings from the environment and social context in which they live. These elements are illustrated in Figure 4.1 which also shows some of the consequences of this model for the practice of medicine and for the practice of other disciplines that work closely with medicine, for example, midwifery.

The medical model clearly has utility in the diagnosis and treatment of ill-health but it also has negative consequences. In its extreme form the model fragments and objectifies the individual, who experiences care from detached professionals who tend to make all the decisions about care.

Organisations which hold the medical model will be organised in ways which enable the treatment of individual parts of the body, in departments and specialities. Health professionals who hold the medical model will provide care which focuses on a particular organ or aspect of the person. For example, the caricature that anyone admitted to a psychiatric unit will receive attention for their mental health problems but any physical illness they have will go largely untreated is familiar.

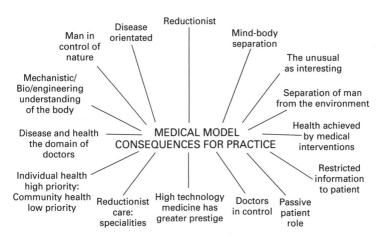

Figure 4.1   *The medical model: consequences for practice*

Kane (1990), rather tongue-in-cheek, describes this as the 'Line-down-the-Middle' theory of nursing, in which psychological and physical health are separated from each other.

Care by midwives who hold the medical model will also demonstrate the features described above. Women will be viewed in terms of their pregnancy rather than as individuals with unique personal and family concerns. Care will be organised around the ability to control the process of childbirth, to reduce professional uncertainty, and women will experience little or no control or choice in their care. Examples of this type of control are found in policies regarding antenatal examinations, ultrasound scans and other tests. Garcia *et al.* (1987) and Garforth and Garcia (1987) describe a study in which they observed the admission of women in labour and identified the restrictive effects of organisational policies on the care experienced by these women. As pregnancy is viewed as a series of stages in this model, rather than a continuous process, care will be divided between different departments and within those departments between different midwives. So there are the antenatal clinic and the antenatal clinic midwives, the labour ward and the labour ward team and divisions in care within these departments as found by Robinson *et al.* (1983).

McKeown (1989) summarises the elements of current medical practice as follows:

> In the broadest sense, the medical role is in the three areas: prevention of disease by personal and non-personal measures; care of patients who require investigation and treatment; and care of the sick who are not thought to need active intervention. Medical interest and resources are focused on the second area and, to a lesser extent, on personal prevention by immunization; the other responsibilities are relatively neglected. (McKeown, 1989, p. 197)

Midwifery care can be summarised as the support of women and families who are well; promoting health and preventative measures and helping in role development, and, in a minority of instances, caring for women who are ill and in need of investigation, treatment and care. Comparison of the purposes of medicine and midwifery indicates that the medical model may not be the most suitable model on which to base midwifery care. The consequences of the medical/obstetric model for care of the childbearing woman are discussed further in Chapter 5.

Another effect of the medical model in the care of the childbearing woman results from the fact that it is a model which is widely held and understood in society. As Vouri and Rimpela (1981) discuss, the utility of this model is one of its strengths. The medical model is the model of care which many women and their families hold. The model indicates certain expectations of care from the viewpoint of the woman as well as the care-giver. The woman will expect the obstetrician, the medical man, to be in control, to be the expert and to make decisions on her behalf. She may therefore feel resentful if asked to make decisions or if she receives care from other health professionals whom she views as less expert than the doctors, for example midwives. She may expect those caring for her to be mainly concerned with the health of the growing fetus and concerned about her health as it affects the fetus. She may then find it difficult to understand why carers, for example midwives, are concerned about her feelings, behaviours or needs which do not relate directly to the pregnancy. She may expect to be cared for by experts at each stage of her pregnancy, for example in the antenatal period, in labour and postnatally. She may then not be concerned that she receives care from different midwives at different stages of her pregnancy, if she has confidence in their expertise. Efforts to achieve continuity of midwives may raise questions in her mind about expertise, particularly in situations where midwives who have worked in one area for a long time are asked to care for women throughout the childbearing process. The medical model thus has consequences for the way women view care, their expectations of care and their view of what is expected of them. Alternative models of care need to be considered in relation to the models held by childbearing women as well as professional groups.

Any alterations in the model of care held by professional groups, for example midwives, or policymakers, such as that proposed in the Expert Committee report (Department of Health, 1993a), will need to be discussed and shared with all other professional groups and, most importantly, with the women with whom services should be developed. The action approach to organisations (Chapter 3) indicates that fundamental change from the medical model which currently forms the basis for much maternity care will require attention at many different points if real change in the organisation of maternity services is to be achieved.

BONDING: A REAPPRAISAL OF THEORY

Models and theories are adopted in practice for a range of reasons and the development and adoption of the theory of bonding provides an illustration of this process. The discussion about bonding is included to illustrate the need to ask questions about theories, to undertake research to demonstrate the validity of a theory and the need to examine the wider effects of a particular theory on the childbearing woman and her family.

Maternal–infant bonding is for many today an almost unquestioned theory, almost a fact of life, and a major area of concern for many midwives caring for women after the birth of their baby (Salariya, 1990). Essentially the theory about maternal–infant 'bonding' is based upon the observation of sensitive periods in their offspring in some species or subspecies of animals and birds which are crucial for the establishment of a care bond between, for example, the bird and its offspring. If the sensitive period is disrupted in some way then the maternal bird does not care for her offspring.

Bonding between the human mother and her baby is said to rest crucially upon immediate or early contact between the mother and her baby and a similar sensitive period is postulated: *if* the mother and baby are together during this sensitive period *then* bonding will occur. Failure to 'bond' has been blamed for difficulties children experience later in learning; as a contributory factor in antisocial behaviour, child abuse and many other ills faced by society (Eyer, 1993).

A number of authors including Richards (1984), MacFarlane (1984) and Eyer (1993) provide critiques of the background to bonding research, the details of the research methods used and the social context of the research. The following discussion is based largely on Eyer (1993): *Mother–Infant Bonding. A Scientific Fiction.*

Interest in bonding was preceded by many years of observation of, and research into, maternal deprivation experienced by orphaned children in institutions and the reactions of children admitted to hospitals which restricted parents from having contact with their children. This work is associated with many child psychologists, including Anna Freud and John Bowlby. More recently, evidence of the effects of extreme contact deprivation have been provided from the orphanages and hospitals in Rumania and other countries in Eastern Europe.

The first research on bonding was published by Kennell and Klaus in the early 1970s. These paediatric researchers studied 28 single women from low-income families and their babies. Fourteen of these pairs had extra periods of contact with their baby in the first three days and fourteen pairs experienced the then-usual hospital regime in which the babies spent the majority of their time in the nursery away from their mothers. Eyer (1993) reviews the criticisms of this research, which includes the failure to follow accepted research principles. Later research discussed has also failed to to amply demonstrate a relationship between early contact and later strengths or difficulties in either the maternal–child relationship or other social behaviours and has failed to demonstrate the existence of a sensitive period in the human maternal–infant relationship. The research evidence, in short, does not support the view that there is a sensitive period for the formation of the maternal–infant relationship which, if not achieved at this time will lead to the long-term failure of the formation of this relationship.

However, the suggestion that there might be such a period in the formation of maternal–infant relationships was a useful weapon for those who were trying to humanise restrictive regimes then current in maternity units. In her discussion, Eyer (1993) focuses on the ways in which knowledge is adopted and used by society to deal with aspects of life that are perceived to present problems. She comments:

> The disparity between the legitimacy of research evidence and its widespread acceptance can be explained only by probing more deeply into the unquestioned assumptions with which the scientific community was operating. (Eyer, 1993, p. 46)

There were also wider reasons prevalent in the wider society, beyond the efforts to improve care in maternity units, which Eyer (1993) argues encouraged the acceptance of a sensitive period and bonding in the maternal–infant relationship, although this notion conflicted with the research findings. Social reasons for the widespread acceptance of the notion of bonding which Eyer (1993) discusses include the need for society to control women, to keep women at home and out of the labour market. In maternity care, bonding provided a scientific rationale for the need to keep mothers and babies together and to humanise obstetric units. Bonding also provided greater power to health professionals involved in care of the mother and baby through the medicalisation of the process of attachment. Women would have to be helped by professionals 'to bond', to deal with the problems of 'failure to bond' and could be criticised by health professionals if they showed a lack of willingness 'to bond'. Bonding therefore provided a strong motivation to organisational change and the further development of professional power over childbirth (Arney, 1982) (see Chapters 3 and 5). Eyer (1993) suggests that for these reasons the concept of bonding, a theoretical idea unsupported by research evidence, was readily accepted and promoted in the care of the childbearing woman.

This is a view supported by Richards (1984) who, while commending the changes in hospital regimes, comments that the price of those changes may have been too high. Many parents have been convinced by the notion of bonding and become distressed and concerned if they were unable, for whatever reasons, to spend time with their baby immediately after birth. This may then result in long-term guilt reactions which have been induced by a theory which is not supported by research evidence. Another danger of the widespread acceptance of the notion of a sensitive period in human beings identified by MacFarlane (1984) is the way the notion becomes an explanation for all family disruption and breakdown and an excuse for lack of action by health professionals:

> On the other hand, overemphasis on the concept of bonding as separate from the total developing relationship between parents and their children from conception onwards may be dangerous, because for doctors and other health workers it may become a cure-all for the effects of poverty, family disruption and psychosocial factors – problems for which there may be far more appropriate forms of intervention. (MacFarlane, 1984, p. 61)

Eyer (1993) concludes with a call for the term bonding to be discarded and for an acknowledgement that relationships are formed of many different elements:

> strong relationships require many ingredients; they seldom endure automatically. Constructive relationships involve love, understanding, trust, time, money, sharing, giving, stimulating and inspiring. Discarding the word *bonding* would force us to notice that children are not merely putty in our hands. (Eyer, 1993, p. 199).

Bonding provides an example of the adoption in practice, in care of the childbearing woman, of a theory from another discipline, the study of sensitive periods in some animal species. This example suggests that theory may be adopted and used for a wide variety of reasons – in this case, the need to change organisational practices. In other cases, theory may be adopted to maintain the power and control of one profession over another or over lay groups. The development and use of theory is not value-free but dependent on values held by different groups within society. This examination of the theory of bonding suggests that it is necessary to question and examine the values underpinning any theory.

HEALTH FOR ALL

The model of Health for All, propounded by the World Health Organization since 1978, has not had a great deal of overt support and promotion within health care in the United Kingdom, let alone in midwifery practice (World Health Organization, 1981). It is a model which enables the focus of care to be on the woman, her family and community and which also provides a means of communication with midwives in other countries. While discussion of this model has not been overt, the covert influence of the model in much government policy in relation to maternity services is significant and it has important consequences for midwifery care.

The medical model, as shown above, is focused on the individual and the disease process and has wide influence at the levels of patient care, government policy and in the field of international health. In contrast, the Health for All model focuses on the community, the environment and the wider strategies needed to support and promote health in its widest sense. The Health for All model was developed by the World Health Organization and stated in the Declaration of Alma-Ata in 1978 (WHO, 1981). This then is a model which has been developed at the level of international society but which seeks to bring about radical change in the structures of health care organisations, the wider views in societies regarding health, the attitudes of health care practitioners and members of the community and in the provision of health care.

The underlying philosophy of this conceptual model is stated in the Declaration and is a statement of support for the WHO definition of health:

> The Conference strongly reaffirms that health, which is a state of complete physical, mental and social wellbeing, and not merely the absence of disease or infirmity, is a fundamental human right and that the attainment of the highest possible level of health is a most important worldwide social goal whose realisation requires the action of many other social and economic sectors in addition to the health sector. (World Health Organization, 1988, p. 7)

The Declaration goes on to emphasise the need for other sectors of society to be involved in health care and identifies primary health care as the focus for health care and the means of achieving the goal of Health for All by the year 2000.

Ewles and Simnett (1992) identify five themes in the Health for All movement:

> reducing inequalities in health;
> positive health through health promotion and disease prevention;
> community participation;
> cooperation between health authorities, local authorities and others with an impact on health;
> a focus on primary health care as the main basis of the health care system. (Ewles and Simnett, 1992, p. 13)

Primary health care is described as the vehicle for health, a view which is in sharp contrast to that of the medical model where the focus is on the provision of specialised, hospital-based services (Macdonald, 1993). Primary health care is defined as follows:

Primary health care is essential health care based on practical, scientifically sound and socially acceptable methods and technology made universally accessible to individuals and families in the community through their full participation and at a cost that the community and country can afford to maintain at every stage of their development in the spirit of self-reliance and self-determination. It forms an integral part both of the country's health system, of which it is the central function and main focus, and of the overall social and economic development of the community. It is the first level of contact of individuals, the family and community with the national health system bringing health as close as possible to where people live and work, and constitutes the first element of a continuing health care process. (WHO, 1988, p. 8).

The model of Health for All and the definition of primary health care include five concepts (WHO, 1988):

1. Equity of provision of health care by universal coverage of the population with care provided according to need;
2. Services should be promotive, preventive, curative and rehabilitative, that is, services meeting these different types of need should be provided in an integrated way (all services being in one place) – the supermarket approach to health care as it is described in Zimbabwe;
3. Services should be effective, culturally acceptable, affordable and manageable, that is, services should meet needs in ways that are acceptable to the population and services should be monitored and managed effectively;
4. Communities should be involved in the development, provision and monitoring of services, that is, the provision of health care is the responsibility of the whole community and health is seen as a factor contributing to overall community development;
5. Inter-sectoral collaboration, that is, that health and health care are not dependent on health services alone but affected by such factors as housing, environmental pollution, food supply and advertising methods.

These concepts describe the underlying principles and should be observable in health services. In addition to these concepts, eight areas for action have been identified for achieving Health for All via primary health care. These eight areas are:

1. Education about prevailing health problems and methods of preventing and controlling them.
2. Promotion of food supply and proper nutrition.
3. An adequate supply of safe water and basic sanitation.
4. Maternal and child health, including family planning.
5. Immunisation against infectious diseases.
6. Prevention and control of endemic diseases.
7. Appropriate control of common diseases and injuries.
8. Provision of essential drugs. (Morley *et al.*, 1989, p. x).

Maternal and child health is identified within this model as one of the key areas for action to achieve Health for All but it can also be seen that the five underlying concepts and the areas for action all have an impact on the care of the childbearing women, as shown in Figure 4.2.

The Health for All conceptual model identifies a whole range of areas in which action can be taken. The actions taken by individuals, organisations or governments who are seeking to implement this model will result in actions which are very different to those undertaken by individuals, organisations or governments holding a medical model. Some suggested consequences for action in relation to maternity services are shown in Figure 4.2. Consequences for action for maternity care involving the application of the five concepts to each action area can also be described. For example, what are the consequences for action of applying the five concepts to promotion of food supply and proper nutrition for childbearing women?

In Britain there has been little overt discussion of the Health for All model and it may be criticised, for example on economic grounds, as being unattainable or altruistic (Andreano, 1993). Some of the problems of applying this model in health care practice are as follows:

1. Community participation, with an emphasis on self-care, is inconsistent with the patterns of conventional health services delivery and the predominant attitudes of health professionals.
2. There is little or no precedent for multisectoral co-operation in the management and control of health problems.
3. All too frequently the extension of health service coverage to underserved and at-risk groups is not accomplished because health professionals do not deliver health care to such groups but rather wait for them to approach a health care facility or service. (World Health Organization, 1989, p. 4).

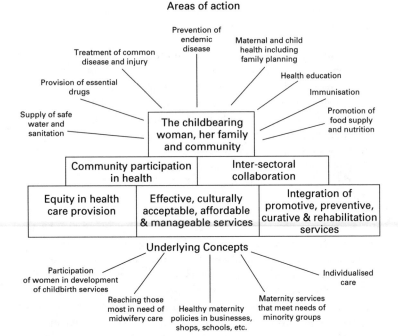

Figure 4.2   *The Health for All model: consequences for practice*

These are serious problems and indicate that if health services are to be reorientated to primary health care and based on the five concepts described above then great changes will be needed in the education of health care practitioners, in the organisation of services and in the involvement of individuals in their own health care.

Evidence for changes in line with the Health for All model can be found world-wide, including Britain (WHO, 1988). In relation to care of the childbearing woman the most important world-wide challenge is to reduce the maternal mortality rate from its current estimated level of 500 000 per year (Kwast, 1993; Maclean, 1993). Consideration of the concepts and areas of action for Health for All indicates that the provision of safe care for women in their homes and local communities has the greatest potential to reduce this number of deaths. One of the initiatives aimed at improving the care that women receive in their communities is the initiative to improve the knowledge of traditional birth attendants (TBAs). TBAs are the people who are with the majority of women during the childbirth process. This initiative provides training for TBAs and training of those, including midwives, who train TBAs (WHO, 1992).

The Facts for Life initiative seeks, again through education, to improve maternal health by bringing ten simple health-education messages to communities and individuals throughout the world (UNICEF, 1990a, 1990b).

For example, the three messages relating to maternal health are applicable throughout the world:

1. The health of both women and children can be significantly improved by spacing births at least two years apart, by avoiding pregnancies before the age of 18, and by limiting the total number of pregnancies to four.
2. To reduce the dangers of childbearing, all pregnant women should go to a health worker for pre-natal care and all births should be assisted by a trained person.
3. For the first few months of a baby's life, breastmilk *alone* is the best possible food and drink. Infants need other foods, 'n addition to breastmilk, when they are four-to-six months old. (UNICEF, 1990a, p. xiii)

International, national and local targets also indicate the adoption of this model in policy. For example, of the 38 European Targets for Health for All, over half relate either directly or indirectly to achieving changes which will contribute to maternal and child health. Target 8 is directly concerned with reducing maternal mortality in the European region but targets relating to lifestyles (for example, Target 17: Health-Damaging Behaviour); the environment (for example, Target 25: Working Environment); appropriate care (for example, Target 31: Ensuring Quality of Care); and to research and health development support all have implications for the development of maternity services (WHO, 1985b).

In Britain the Health of the Nation consultative document identified as an objective: 'To reduce preventable death and ill-health in pregnant women, infants and children' (Department of Health, 1991, p. 77). Following the consultation process, maternal health was not included as a key area (NHS Management Executive, 1992) but the consultative document shows how the action areas from the international model of Health for All can be translated to the British context. At the regional level, for example in Wales, Maternal and Early Child Health is one of the health gain areas that is being targeted (Welsh Health Planning

Forum, 1991). One example of the maternal and early child health targets is concerned with breast-feeding:

> By 1997, each district should increase the number of women breast feeding for 6 weeks to at least 75% and reduce the pattern of social disparity in breast feeding rates across the population. (Welsh Health Planning Forum, 1991, p. 11)

Breast-feeding is a personal activity which is influenced by family and social attitudes as well as professional advice and support. Reference to Figures 4.2 and 3.2 indicate areas that might need attention if this ambitious target is to be achieved. For example, policies and facilities will be needed which support breast-feeding as well as attitudes in society which encourage and expect women to breast-feed. Achievement of this target can be seen to be linked to some of the areas for action identified in the Health for All model, including promotion of nutrition, prevention of endemic disease and maternal and child health, among others.

The application of this model can also be seen in the Winterton Report (House of Commons Health Committee, 1992) and documents from professional bodies such as the Royal College of Midwives (The RCM, 1991). The Expert Committee Report (Department of Health, 1993a) emphasises the establishment of local, community-based midwifery teams enabling women to experience choice, continuity and control. Such services are, of necessity, an integral part of primary health care, as indicated in the Health for All model and supported by the Safe Motherhood Initiative:

> The taskforce felt also that the maternal health team could not be separated conceptually from the primary health care (PHC) team. Rather it must be either identical to it or a subset of it depending on the circumstances in the country, region or district. (WHO, 1990, p. 6)

So, it can be seen that these reports, which support the establishment of the local midwifery team, reflect the wider principles of the Health for All model, with its emphasis on locally-based services and primary health care as the central focus of all health care. These reports also acknowledge another key concept in the Health for All model: that primary health care is more than care provided by health professionals and must therefore be based in or as close to the woman's home as possible. Thus, adoption of this model in practice has significant implications for the organisation of maternity services (which can be seen to be adopting this model with the establishment of community-based midwifery teams), education of midwives and others, and the day-to-day practice of midwives.

PARTICIPATION IN CARE

In this final section one of the concepts of the Health for All model, participation, is considered. There is much rhetoric about continuity, choice and control for women within maternity services and extensive change is proposed and is beginning to occur in the structure of those services. The reality of participation has consequences for practitioners and childbearing women which are implicit in midwifery teamwork, midwifery-led units and in other innovations.

Earlier in this chapter the consequences of the medical model for care of the childbearing woman were discussed and in Chapter 5 the medical model is contrasted with the model of pregnancy as a normal life-event (see Figure 5.1). Since probably the sixteenth century there has been a growing tension between these two models as the scientific basis of medicine has become better understood. Prior to the increase in scientific knowledge the personal knowledge of women who were pregnant and women who helped women in labour was respected and valued and women were active participants in all aspects of their care (Ehrenreich and English, 1973). However, with the growth of medical knowledge and abstract knowledge, the knowledge of the woman about herself and her own body became devalued. As illustrated in Figure 4.1, one of the consequences of the medical model is the characterisation of the patient or childbearing woman as a passive recipient of care rather than a co-partner in her care.

In the field of maternity care there is a long history of resistance by women to lack of involvement in their care and initiation of movements and other activities which seek to increase that participation (Sullivan and Weitz, 1988). In Britain national organisations such as the Association for Improvements in Maternity Services (AIMS) and The National Childbirth Trust (NCT) which represent the views of child-bearing women (as well as providing other activities) have been in existence for many years. The influence of these bodies can be seen in the evidence that they produce for government committees (see for example AIMS, 1992) and resources that they produce to help in the implementation of change (see, for example, National Childbirth Trust, 1993). At the level of the individual, the use of birth plans which has developed since the late 1970s is one example of attempts to involve women and their families more centrally in their care (Carty and Tier, 1989).

More widely in the health services, the introduction of the Patients
Charter (HMSO, 1992) has had a significant effect on placing the
patient (the individual) at the centre of health service concern. In maternity care recent reports have emphasised the need for services to be
women-centred, to make information available to women and to be
concerned with the local community:

> The services provided should recognise the special characteristics of
> the population they are designed to serve. They should also be attrac-
> tive and accessible to all women, particularly those who may be least
> inclined to use them.
>
> Information about the local maternity services should be readily
> available within the community....
>
> The woman and, if she wishes, her partner, should be encouraged
> to be closely involved in the planning of her care. (Department of
> Health, 1993a, p. 5)

Government policy, strongly influenced by consumer pressure from
organisations seeking to improve care of the childbearing woman (as
well as by economic pressures and professional pressure), now emphasises the need to involve women in their care at the level of the individual and at the level of service provision, for example in the monitoring
of service contracts (Department of Health, 1993a, p. 61). This consumer or community involvement in health/maternity care has thus
arisen, in part, from consumer pressure for higher standards in maternity services.

This pressure for increased participation would not have arisen if
women were satisfied with the extent to which they were involved in
care and in the development of services. The medical model, discussed
above, restricts the participation of the woman in her own care and es-
tablishes patterns of expectations and interaction between obstetricians,
midwives and childbearing women. The organisational structures, discussed in Chapter 3, also constrain the type of involvement that women
may have or the type of care that midwives may provide. Attitudes,
stereotypes and education may also limit the extent to which midwives
are able or willing to involve women in care (Bowler, 1993).
Participation of women in care involves challenge to professional authority, reduction in the distance that some health professionals try to
establish between themselves and those they care for and sharing of
knowledge and reduction in power, if knowledge is power (McCrea and
Crute, 1991). It is a challenge to the image of the 'professional'
midwife discussed in Chapter 5. Participation (in the form of establishing good relationships), as McCrea and Crute (1991) found, is also

dependent on the confidence that midwives have in their own role and the extent to which women appreciate the skills and knowledge of midwives.

Participation can be considered on two levels: the level of the individual woman–midwife interaction and at the level of the community. On the level of the individual woman–midwife interaction the inclusion or exclusion of the concept of participation in the picture of care held by the individual midwife will affect the extent to which the care provided by that midwife involves the woman (in the context of the organisation within which the midwife is working). Some of the models for midwifery practice emphasise the involvement of the woman in her care. Wiedenbach (1967) goes so far as to imply that care is dependent on the recognition by the woman of a Need-for-Help, while Lehrman (1981) identified participation in care (participative care) as one of the eight components of a model of nurse-midwifery practice in antenatal care.

Littlewood (1989) contrasts the lay and professional understanding of symptoms and discusses the different meanings that a women may ascribe to symptoms in a description of care of a woman with signs of toxaemia (pre-eclampsia). For reasons that are not made clear, Littlewood (1989) uses the term nurse when discussing the activities of midwives in this article. Using theory from the anthropological literature, Littlewood (1989) comments on the need to understand the 'patient's own model of disease causation' (p. 228) if services are to become actively patient-centred. Understanding of the model of health or ill-health held by an individual woman requires the active involvement of the woman in her care and attention by the midwife to the social context of the woman's life. Littlewood (1989) comments that the bio-medical approach involves collection of information about signs and symptoms, including raised blood pressure and proteinurea on the basis of which a diagnosis is made and care prescribed. For the woman herself the meaning of the signs and symptoms is based on her knowledge and ways of interpreting the world. Littlewood (1989) suggests the woman may ascribe the raised blood pressure to having worked too hard or may see it as a punishment, or it may not be considered important but something which 'runs in the family'. The author proposes a model of care which has at its centre the concept of the woman's perception of her health and is termed the Generalised Nursing Model. Assessment areas include: 'How would the treatment of the disturbance be effected within the person's peer group and family? Are there any rituals usually surrounding this problem?' (Littlewood, 1989, p. 227). Evaluation of care includes the need to assess: 'Does the person feel healed?' and 'Has the lay cause of the disorder been understood and discussed?' (p. 227). The midwife who holds a model of care which includes the need to assess the woman's understanding of her symptoms will, of necessity, involve the woman in her care.

Such a model of care is required if the needs of the individual woman, which are rooted in her social and cultural experience, are to be understood and met and if the proposed first principle of the maternity services is to be achieved:

> The woman must be the focus of maternity care. She should be able to feel that she is in control of what is happening to her and able to make decisions about her care, based on her needs, having discussed matters fully with the professionals involved. (Department of Health, 1993a, p. 9)

That this is not the model which is commonly experienced by women during childbearing is illustrated in two surveys. Salford Community Health Council (1992) found that 27 per cent of first-time mothers (sample 66) and 44 per cent of women having subsequent births (sample 84) felt they had no choice in the place of delivery and lacked information about such choices. There were similar findings in a sample of 1271 women who completed a questionnaire distributed by the National Childbirth Trust (Newburn, 1993):

> More than half the women, 56%, said they were offered no choice about where they might have their baby and who might be responsible for their care, and a massive 94% said they were given no written information about alternative places of birth and who could provide care. (Newburn, 1993, p. 20)

These examples suggest that the women who completed these two surveys were receiving care which was not based on a model which included the concept of participation. Littlewood's (1989) description of the need to understand the meanings ascribed by women to events combined with the results of these surveys indicates the need for the model of care held by the individual midwife to include the concept of participation if the woman is to be an active participant in her care.

However, as discussed in Chapter 3, the care experienced by a woman is not only dependent on the attitudes of individual midwives. The quotation above (Department of Health, 1993a) illustrates government policy, one aspect of the knowledge and attitudes to maternity care in the wider society (see Figure 3.1), which supports the provision of woman-centred services. The pervasive nature of the medical model, with its associated attitudes which are widely held in society, means that this recent change in the attitudes of policymakers is counteracted by attitudes in society and among individuals which have resulted in the dependence of members of the community on medical and other health professionals. This is in contrast to the attitudes in the wider society in the Netherlands (see Chapter 3) where participation and the taking of personal responsibility, for example, in homebirth within a structured system of needs assessment, is a more widely-held attitude.

Organisations also have significant effects on participation at the level of the woman–midwife encounter. The extent to which the concept of participation is included in the model of care supported by organisations providing maternity care will affect the extent to which the woman is involved in her care and in the development of services. Organisational attitudes are demonstrated, for example, in policies and procedures which may inhibit individualised care through reference to safety and support of practices which are not research-based (Garforth and Garcia, 1987). Organisational strategies which have been developed to increase participation include the setting-up of team midwifery schemes (see for example Titcombe, 1991), the introduction of women-held records, improved information and standard-setting initiatives (Department of Health, 1993b). Concern has been expressed that some attempts at involving (in this case) patients in care may be seen as attempts to increase compliance with prescribed care rather than increasing the autonomy of the patient (Brearley, 1990). Similarly consumer satisfaction surveys, a means by which an organisation may involve consumers in commenting on services, run the risk of being token exercises which generally produce positive responses (Warrier, 1991).

The extent to which other health professionals hold models of care which inhibit the concept of participation, such as the medical model, will also influence the extent to which midwives are able to involve women in care.

Achieving participation in care, by women and by the community within which they live, presents challenges to professional power and models of practice while requiring midwives and other health professionals to exercise new skills which help women get involved in their care. Achieving participation may therefore not be quite as easy as it first appears. As discussed above, in recent reports on maternity services two types of participation are identified: participation in personal care planning and participation in the monitoring of services, but other types of participation are also described in the wide literature on the involvement of individuals and communities in health care. These forms of participation may need different types of support and encouragement by midwives. Brearley (1990) identifies the key aspects of the literature on patient participation as:

self-help: active patient involvement in care;
demedicalisation or deprofessionalisation: substitution of lay for professional care;
democratisation: involvement of consumers in social policy decisions in the field of health care. (Brearley, 1990, pp. 2–3)

These aspects of the concept indicate that participation is understood to involve increasing the ability of individuals to care for themselves and their families and to be actively involved in their care. Such increased activity implies education and advice on care – for example, in antenatal clinics or on the postnatal ward. The substitution of lay for professional care may be seen in the attendance of women at classes run by the National Childbirth Trust (although the concept of professional volunteer may be relevant here) or the potential that lay people have for meeting needs of women in the early postnatal period. Democratisation and involvement of women in service development can be seen in the potential of Maternity Services Liaison Committees.

At the community level there are also different interpretations of participation or community involvement in health as it is described in the Health for All model (see above). Community participation in health is based on the long tradition of development work in other areas such as agriculture and self-reliance movements (Macdonald, 1993). Oakley (1989) identifies two main approaches to community involvement in health in the literature: '*awareness* and *understanding* of health and health problems; ....access to information and knowledge about health services programmes and projects'(Oakley, 1989, p. 13). These two approaches to community involvement in health are significantly different. Much of the discussion of participation, above, can be seen to relate to the second description of involvement in health, where women are provided with improved information and access to services, important goals in services which are lacking in these respects, as indicated in the survey results presented above.

Oakley (1989) describes the differences in these approaches as follows:

The first interpretation lays stress on building up communities' awareness and understanding of the problems of health development and the causes of poor health as the basis for their future active involvement in health development. The second interpretation emphasizes that communities must have direct access to specific information and knowledge about health service programmes and projects as a pre-condition for becoming involved in health activities designed and to be directed by others. (Oakley, 1989, pp. 13–14)

The first description is inherently more radical than the second, as it suggests the potential of community participation in health to address inequalities in health. These descriptions illustrate the point that Oakley (1989) reiterates, that there is no single interpretation of the concept of community participation in health. These different interpretations do, however, indicate that community involvement in health or participation may operate at different levels. These different levels have been described by Rifkin (1990) who identified five levels of participation in an analysis of maternal and childhealth services. The following discussion of levels of participation is based on Rifkin (1990), pp. 12–15:

Level 1 Participation in the benefits of a programme: at this level people receive services in a passive way and their only involvement is in attending for the service, for example, attending an antenatal clinic.

Level 2 Participation in the activities of a programme: in these programmes members of the community are active participants but in activities decided by health planners, for example, a woman who has had experience of breast-feeding might be asked to lead a discussion on feeding in an antenatal class.

Level 3 Participation in the implementation of programmes: at this level, members of the local community have managerial responsibility in the programme in addition to participating in the benefits and the activities of the programme. Again the activities are identified by the programme planners rather than the community, but the members of the community: 'make decisions about how these activities are to be run' (Rifkin, 1990, p. 13). This type of participation is illustrated by the work of the Newcastle Community Midwifery Care Project which sought to make midwifery care more accessible from a community base in a deprived area but also sought to increase the self-confidence and self-reliance of members of the community so that an outcome of the project has been involvement of the community at this level of participation:

> Many residents have been helped and are increasingly helping themselves, not least in taking responsibility for the Centre. Initially there was a lot of vandalism, but this has improved as local residents have become involved in the management and running of the building. (Davies and Evans, 1991, p. 110).

Level 4 Participation in programme monitoring and evaluation: at this level the local community is involved in setting standards, monitoring services and making modifications to the objectives of the programme. The work of Maternity Services Liaison Committees is an example of community participation at this level, although Rifkin (1990) comments that this level of participation may be the least commonly experienced, due to the lack of priority given to programme evaluation and the lack of clear programme objectives which makes evaluation very difficult.

Level 5 Participation in planning programmes: at this level people are involved in deciding the health services that are needed, as well as being involved at the preceding levels:

> This is the level at which community participation is the broadest, in both range and depth. It involves members of the community in receiving benefits, in joining in activities, in implementing projects, in evaluating and monitoring programmes, and in making decisions about, and taking responsibility for, programme policy and management. It is the ideal towards which many programmes strive. (Rifkin, 1990, pp. 14–15)

The different levels of participation suggest different roles for health care practitioners, including midwives, for women and members of their families and local communities. At the first level the professional is in charge but the degree of control exercised by professionals gradually reduces to a point at which the community and health professionals are joint providers. Such a different role and participatory relationship with women and the local community means that midwives would need to consider and make adaptations to their personal models of midwifery practice, changes would be needed in midwifery education, and changes would be needed in midwives' inter- and intra-professional relationships to enable them to take responsibility to be full participants with women.

The achievement of participatory care on the level of the individual woman and at the organisational level presents significant challenges which midwifery shares with other areas of health care which are seeking to develop community and individual participation. A World Health Organization study group which examined the issues involved in making these changes comments:

> To date there is not much evidence that the education of health personnel has changed in ways that will allow them to understand and be committed to CIH as part of their professional activities. This is perhaps because CIH touches on the very relationship between health

personnel and their clients and challenges health personnel to question the nature of that relationship (i.e. to move away from the idea of provider/recipient to one of partnership). (World Health Organization, 1991, p. 20)

This discussion has shown that if women are going to experience more participatory care, to have more choice and control, change will be needed in many aspects of maternity care. Change will be needed at the level of society in the model of care of the childbearing woman and this can be seen to be happening (World Health Organization, 1985a; Department of Health, 1993a). Change will be needed in the formal structures of health organisations with devolved decision-making, valuing of staff and their active involvement in decision-making. Health care practitioners who are not encouraged to be active participants in health care organisations are probably less likely to encourage the active participation of women and their families in care. Change will be needed in the attitudes of midwives, who will have to develop those skills which encourage participation. Change will be needed in the expectations of women and their families of the type of interaction they can expect to have with midwives. Change in the attitudes of other health practitioners involved in maternity care is also necessary. Participatory care provided by one group of health practitioners which is not supported by other groups may lead to conflict and uncertainty for the childbearing woman. Making the concept of participation a reality in the care of every childbearing woman requires discussion of the models of pregnancy held by all participants in care and may require modification of some models which result in care which is more controlling than participatory.

Summary

In this chapter four examples of models, theories and concepts which inform the environment of midwifery care have been considered. Each of these has had a significant impact on, or has the potential to have a significant impact on the provision of maternity care. The medical model is long-established and so ingrained within health care organisations that it may sometimes be difficult to appreciate the far-reaching impact it has. The medical model has contributed to restrictive practices in maternity units, one aspect of which was overturned by bonding theory. The research which tested the theory of bonding did not support the evidence of a sensitive period but this discussion showed that models and theories are sometimes adopted despite research findings because of the need to achieve different ends. In contrast to the medical model the impact of the Health for All model has been less obvious but this discussion indicates the significant impact the model has had at the level of policymaking. Consideration of the concepts of the model indicates that it is a model which may have potential in focusing maternity services on health and locating those services within the woman's local community. Participation, one concept of the Health for All model, was discussed in depth as providing an example of the need to define what is actually meant by such familiar concepts. The potential and challenges of participatory care were considered with the changes that would be needed to achieve such care.

Activities

In this chapter it has only been possible to review a small number of the models and theories influencing midwifery practice. The aim of the following activities is to assist in the identification of other models, theories and concepts in midwifery and to consider their influence, and the influence of those reviewed in this chapter, on practice.

1 In addition to those areas listed at the beginning of this chapter, identify disciplines, models, theories and concepts which inform the environment of midwifery care.

2 Take one of the models, theories or concepts identified in Activity 1 and describe the consequences that it has for practice.

3 Considering your own practice, how does the medical model influence your care?

4 What changes are being made in the maternity services in your area? Identify and describe the concepts and model of maternity care on which these changes are based.

5 Describe incidents from your own practice which were informed by the theory of bonding. What effects has this theory had on your practice?

6 What changes would be needed in the education of midwives if the Health for All model was to be widely adopted in the provision of maternity services?

7 Consider one of the five concepts forming the Health for All model. What consequences does this concept have for midwifery practice?

8 In what ways do women participate in maternity care where you are working?

9 In what ways are you involved as an active participant in the development and evaluation of maternity services? Does your level of

involvement affect your attitude towards involving women in their own care?

10 Describe indicators, in terms which could be measured, that could be used to assess the extent to which women are active participants in their care.

CHAPTER FIVE

Current concepts of midwifery practice

Thus a midwife's most basic responsibility to her clients is to do her utmost to promote comfort, relaxation and peace of mind. Her skills encompass both medical techniques and less concrete abilities to intuit, evoke and channel. Her hands are probably her most precious tools, as she senses, blesses and heals with her touch. The manner in which a midwife assists a birth definitely influences both pleasure and safety. She serves as a mirror, offering appropriate, timely suggestions. She strives continually to reserve judgment and yet speak the truth. (Davis, 1987, p. 7)

INTRODUCTION

In Chapter 4 some models and theories from a range of disciplines which inform the environment of midwifery care and the practice of midwifery were identified. The aim of this chapter is to examine the models and philosophies of care held by midwives as expressed in the midwifery literature. These are the models and theories of midwifery care that will form the actor's (the midwife's) definition of the situation and will influence the action, the care provided (see Figures 3.1 and 3.2). In most cases these models and philosophies are not stated as such but emerge from the writings of these midwives. These models and actions which stem from the models can be described as lying at different points on a continuum between the model of pregnancy as a normal life-event and the obstetric/medical model of pregnancy as only normal in retrospect. This chapter ends with a discussion of that continuum.

Throughout this chapter, as with the whole of the book, the underlying purpose in examining these models, philosophies and theories of care is to consider and question how these different mental pictures influence the care of women during childbearing. What assumptions does each of these models (mental pictures) make about women and childbirth? How does the model affect the assessment information that is collected by the midwife? How does the model influence the participation of the woman in her own care?

This chapter is, of necessity, selective, although the aim has been to present as comprehensive a picture as possible of the thinking about midwifery care which is demonstrated in the British literature.

PICTURES OF MIDWIVES AND MIDWIFERY CARE

The following description of the models of care held by midwives are drawn from books that are available in most midwifery libraries and have therefore influenced the way student midwives and midwives think about midwifery.

Starting with Myles' *Textbook For Midwives*, one of the most influential textbooks in Britain. The description in the Tenth Edition of that book emphasises the professionalism of the midwife:

The British midwife, a highly competent professional woman, is legally licensed as a practitioner of normal obstetrics. During pregnancy she supervises and teaches the expectant mother; throughout labour she makes observations, examinations and decisions on which maternal and fetal life and well-being depend; having delivered the baby she attends to mother and child during the postnatal period. (Myles, 1985, p. 1)

Her education (there is no reference to male midwives) includes 'deep knowledge of the physiological processes of human reproduction being an essential foundation for proficient obstetric practice'. And 'To meet the needs of an enlightened community with improved socio-economic standards the midwife has adopted the wider concepts of obstetric care, for example, sociological, educational and psychological' (Myles, 1985, pp. 1–2).

Myles emphasises the development of clinical skills and craftsmanship: 'One of the assets of the British midwife is her ability as a craftswoman; the tendency in some quarters to denigrate this fundamental faculty is to be deprecated' (Myles, 1985, p. 4). The midwife is placed firmly within the obstetric team: 'It would now be considered a retrograde step for a midwife to take sole charge of an expectant mother, thereby depriving her of the scientific expert care that only the obstetric team can provide' (Myles, 1985, p. 2).

The midwife is also described as a teacher:

This is one of the definitive and most exigent roles of the modern midwife, who by giving appropriate instruction can motivate and prepare prospective mothers to fulfil their reproductive and maternal roles successfully and happily. (Myles, 1985, p. 3)

The midwife is also supportive, although that support is qualified by its professional nature and inverted commas around caring: 'The midwife in a supportive role provides professional companionship and demonstrates a "caring" attitude as an integral part of good obstetric practice' (Myles, 1985, p. 3).

The picture of midwifery that Myles gives concentrates on the practice of the midwife: she is knowledgeable, clinically skilled, a craftswoman, an educator and able to provide support and care.

This professional midwife is essentially oriented towards being a part of the obstetric team and to meeting the needs of the women within (the confines of) the practice of the obstetric team. The actions of the midwife are related to her knowledge base and the organisational role system within which she works. The language of this textbook has been discussed by Leap (1993) and reflects the philosophical stance of the author against 'permissiveness'. Both the overt description of the midwife and the overt and covert description of attitudes held by the author and encouraged in midwives, present an image of a detached professional, working within an obstetric team and obstetric model of care, focusing on skilled physical care with support, counselling and education as necessary.

Modern Obstetrics For Student Midwives (Towler and Butler-Manuel, 1980), on the other hand, gives little idea of how a midwife thinks about practice. In a brief introduction, this book takes an historical approach to an account of the development of midwifery, ending with some of the duties laid on midwives by the Central Midwives Board. The remainder of this book of over 700 pages, is concerned with normal and abnormal aspects of pregnancy and newborn babies and the structure of services. The implication of this textbook, as with many other textbooks for midwives, is that midwifery practice is largely dependent on attaining skills in physical care, as Ball (1987) comments:

My training as a midwife had not given me any information about the psychological processes which underlie transition to motherhood; indeed most midwifery and obstetric textbooks lead one to assume that once the baby is safely born, the mother is instantly able to cope with her new role. The textbooks discuss the physiological processes of the puerperium, the nutritional needs of the infant and something of the formation of maternal–child relationships, but virtually nothing about how to help a woman cope with the varying demands and expectations that mothering brings (Ball, 1987, p. ix).

Beyond this lack of concern with the psychological or sociological these textbooks also provide little insight into the process of 'transition to midwife' and an understanding of how the individual's views, attitudes and knowledge coalesce into a model of midwifery care and practice. In Wiedenbach's phrase, there is no evidence of a 'Summary of Thinking' identifying ideas and insights as well as the development of skills in the practice setting which help the student to identify how they are thinking/modelling midwifery (Nickel *et al.*, 1992). In more recent textbooks the models again have to be deduced rather than being made explicit. This contrasts with American textbooks, which generally commence with one or more chapters considering the philosophies and models of care held by midwives, although the models and theories considered by these American authors to be important for midwifery care are largely drawn from other disciplines rather than from midwifery practice (see Chapter 4; Jensen *et al.*, 1977; Moore, 1983).

In more recent textbooks and articles the philosophies held by the writers are more explicit. The most recent edition of Myles' *Textbook for Midwives* (Bennett and Brown, 1993) emphasises the independent practice of the midwife and the partnership between the midwife and the childbearing woman: 'Midwifery care is a balance between giving care and affirming the woman's ability to care for herself' (Bennett and Brown, 1993, p. 5). The picture painted of the midwife in this book is firmly based on the International Confederation of Midwives' definition of a midwife and includes reference to the midwife being skilled in undertaking and managing midwifery care; in promoting health and communicating; in acting as an independent practitioner in relation to care of women experiencing a normal pregnancy; in working as a member of a team with other health practitioners; in being aware of new knowledge and research findings; in practising within the law and within ethical standards. This textbook lays emphasis on the responsibilities of midwives to maintain their competence, to keep accurate records and to act responsibly in relation to the families for whom they care.

Two additional responsibilities of the midwife are also identified: to the profession and to society. These responsibilities require the midwife to act in a way which preserves standards and to draw: 'midwifery issues to the attention of the public' (Bennett and Brown, 1993, p. 7). In relation to society the midwife is described as being able to identify problems such as poverty, poor housing and racial prejudice and to respond to these issues: 'Her response in such circumstances may be to warn, to mobilise resources or to offer active care' (Bennett and Brown, 1993, p. 8). This description of the midwife identifies a number of concepts which these authors consider should inform the practice of this questioning, independent practitioner who is involved continuously in developing and helping to move midwifery care forward:

> Midwives have a responsibility for the image of their profession. For all to keep moving forward, each individual must be sufficiently committed to play an active role in order to preserve standards and improve care. For some this will mean initiating change or trying experiments, for others it will mean following in the footsteps of the innovators. (Bennett and Brown, 1993, p. 7)

In another recent textbook, which is aimed at examining and demonstrating the theoretical, research base of midwifery practice, Silverton (1993) states that the role of the midwife, and by implication the model of practice held by the midwife, is central to the book, *The Art and Science of Midwifery*. A detailed description of the historical development of the role of the midwife and a critique of the erosion of the role through the medicalisation of birth and the effects of the nursing culture on midwifery practice are provided. The discussion highlights the central place of the midwife in the care of the woman experiencing a normal birth and a number of schemes are discussed which enable midwives to utilise all their skills. This midwife's philosophy of care is clearly shown in this extract:

> If midwifery is to prosper it must foster articulate, intelligent and perceptive midwives who can represent midwifery to other professional groups, government agencies and to the general public. Their practice must be based upon sound research, giving the midwife the ability to argue the rationale for her management from a sound theoretical base. Midwives must be responsive to the needs of mothers and families. (Silverton, 1993, p. 15)

Page (1993), in an article entitled 'Redefining The Midwife's Role: Changes needed in practice', describes the attributes that midwives will need to care for women in the late twentieth century. The midwife should be 'with the woman', a skilled clinician, knowledgeable about the latest scientific research, a professional practitioner, a skilled companion and: 'In using clinical judgment and making clinical decisions, the midwife needs a foundation of clear concepts, theories, scientific evidence and clinical experience' (Page, 1993, p. 23).

Seven aims for midwifery services over the next five years are outlined by Page (1993) who comments that a process of incremental change will be needed to achieve these targets. Examination indicates the underlying concepts implicit in the targets. These include: respect for the individual; participation in care; continuity; knowledgeable practice; measurement of outcomes. These concepts may be applied to the type of care experienced by the woman and the type of care practised by the midwife: see Table 5.1.

Table 5.1 *Nationwide aims for Page's five year strategy for development of midwifery services*

---

1. Continuity of carer and continuity of care throughout the pregnancy.
2. A named midwife to serve as primary contact in the health care service (ideally the same midwife who provides continuity of care).
3. A practitioner the woman knows and has a positive relationship with to care for her in labour and for the birth of her baby (ideally the named midwife).
4. The availability of midwifery-led care for low-risk families who choose it.
5. The ability to provide women and their families with appropriate information about the relative benefits of particular treatments and approaches to care.
6. An organisational culture which explicitly values the rights of women to choose and control their own care.
7. Effective approaches to audit and evaluation of changes in practice and in the organisation.

(Table 1, Page, 1993, p. 23; reproduced with the permission of the *British Journal of Midwifery*)

One of the incremental changes that will be needed if midwives are to achieve these targets is further discussion of the concepts underlying midwifery practice, examination through research of the interrelationships between concepts and development of shared theory on which to build towards the targets.

Page (1993) is essentially arguing for the re-establishment of the practice of midwives as independent, autonomous practitioners, a concept which has been eroded over many years, as illustrated by Myles (1985) above. The reality of midwifery care is, in some cases, markedly different from the type of care and the type of midwife Page (1993) proposes for the care of women in the next century. Hunt and Symonds (in press), for example, provide an illuminating discussion of the context and character of midwifery practice.

Walker (1991) illustrates one midwife's experience of the reality of midwifery practice in the 1990s. Having entered midwifery with high expectations of independent practice and autonomy, she found that the care provided by midwives was restricted by medical policies, the under-utilisation of midwives' skills, constraints imposed by the midwifery management system and the attitude of some women who perceive medical care to be of higher value than care provided by midwives. She suggests that there is an inertia within the profession of midwifery which is comfortable with a limited role, which is nearer to that of the obstetric nurse than the midwife, and which is comfortable within a hierarchical management system, which in itself limits responsibility and autonomy. Walker (1991) describes these concepts from her own experience but it is probable that these are concepts of practice that are held by many midwives working within organisations providing maternity care, although this attitude to midwifery care is rarely expressed in midwifery literature. Evidence of the experience of care from midwives operating within a model of restricted practice is more often found in literature describing the experience of care from the perspective of the childbearing woman (discussed below).

In other books on midwifery practice, the values, attitudes, beliefs and models of midwifery care held are seen as central to the person of the midwife and the way that women are cared for by midwives. These books start from the proposition that the midwife needs to understand herself or himself before caring for others. Again, although not identified as 'models of midwifery' (and possibly some of these authors would balk at this term) these descriptions provide a picture of the elements (concepts) that make up midwifery care.

Inch (1989) summarises the type of care that women seek:

> a personal, continuous relationship with their midwife throughout pregnancy, labour and the postnatal period, so that they had the opportunity to establish a relationship of trust. They wanted privacy, a relaxed and optimistic attitude to the process of labour, support, encouragement and exploration. (Inch, 1989, p. 71)

It is this personal, loving relationship between woman and midwife which is emphasised, for example, by Flint (1989) and Davis (1987). As Inch comments: 'All these things (that women seek) come almost automatically if the woman and her midwife can establish a personal, continuing relationship' (Inch, 1987, p. 71).

Descriptions by these midwives present a common picture of women, health, the environment and midwifery practice and emphasise the need for midwives to know themselves. The individuality of each woman is central to these pictures and midwifery care is oriented to understanding each women and her needs. This understanding enables the midwife to support the woman and develop her self-confidence – one of the overall aims of midwifery care as described by these authors – and to detect changes from the norm occurring to that woman:

'Perhaps the most important way to increase someone's confidence is to listen to them and to show respect towards them, what they have to say, their culture, their ideas and their customs' (Flint, 1989, p. 17).

> By giving thorough pre-natal care, the midwife becomes so familiar with each client that she will be quickly alerted to any deviation from the normal. The birth is the finishing touch to a carefully developed relationship including care on physical, emotional and intellectual levels. (Davis, 1987, p. 5)

Health in these books is described in social, psychological and physical terms. While there is great concern for the physical well-being of the mother and baby (possibly accentuated by the close, friendship relationship advocated) the social and psychological aspects of childbearing are highlighted. For example, Flint (1989) describes ways in which women can be helped to feel more at home and therefore more relaxed in the birth room by wearing their own clothes and having music or photographs with them that are important to them. This model, which identifies the woman as an individual, has consequences for action which is aimed at understanding (by listening and observing) and meeting the individual needs of the woman. If individuality and providing support to maintain the self-image of the woman are not part of the mental picture held by the midwife then actions can be routine and lack attention to the psychological growth of the woman.

This view of the woman requires an assessment of the individual's unique environment, including family relationships, social support, community and other factors, and for the midwife to work in partnership with the woman to address her needs (Ackerman, 1980).

But most importantly these books provide a clear picture of the midwife (which is in sharp contrast to the limited images in some textbooks, e.g. Towler and Butler (1980); Myles (1985)). These books emphasise the need for midwives to know themselves, to take care of themselves and to allow themselves to continue to grow. Davis (1987) comments: 'A midwife's prime offering to others is her uniqueness, her individuality and independent perspective. And in order to keep this alive it must be nourished.' (Davies, 1987, p. 183).

In the title of her book, *Sensitive Midwifery*, Flint (1989) identifies this self-knowledge; people cannot be sensitive unless they know themselves:

> To work as a midwife is stressful, because to work effectively and sensitively, the midwife gives so much of herself, and she becomes so involved with and such a part of the family with which she is

involved. To enable her to be a fount of such strength, a source of so much comfort, she herself must have support and cherishing. (Flint, 1989, p. 1)

Flint (1989) describes different ways for midwives to be supported and cherished but also discusses the lack of support and cherishing that some midwives may experience, particularly in hierarchical organisations, and the consequences this will have on their behaviour to each other and to the women and families with whom they are involved (see Chapter 3).

This caring, self-aware, assertive midwife contrasts with the rather detached, obstetric-oriented, passive midwife found in some midwifery textbooks (Ackerman, 1986) and with the practical experience of midwifery described by Walker (1991). While not stated overtly as models of midwifery practice these books (and many others) illustrate the process that midwives have been going through in thinking about and describing their beliefs, knowledge and values: in constructing their models of practice.

PHILOSOPHIES OF MIDWIFERY CARE

A philosophy, as discussed in Chapter 2, is 'an explicit statement about what you believe and about what values you hold' (Pearson and Vaughan, 1986, p. 8).

During the past ten years, most maternity units and teams of midwives have made explicit the philosophies underpinning the organisation of the unit and the care provided there. This concern with clearly stated philosophies was partly stimulated by the publication of the Maternity Services Advisory Committee reports (1982, 1984, 1985) which have had very wide impact both in practice and education (see, for example, Distance Learning Centre, 1992). These reports contain aims, policy statements, areas for action and checklists which all demonstrate the underlying philosophy of the Committee. For example, the aim of antenatal care indicates that the model of care proposed includes concepts relating to support, health promotion, education and role development:

> To ensure as far as possible the health and wellbeing of the woman and unborn child. Pregnancy and childbirth represent a physical, psychological and social change for the prospective parents, particularly the woman, and antenatal care should provide support and guidance at this time and help them prepare for parenthood. (Maternity Services Advisory Committee, 1982, p. 1)

And in labour the concept of participation is addressed in one of the checklist items that reinforces the participation of the parents and staff in determining care: 'C2. Are the views of parents, whether expressed individually or collectively, and of staff fully considered when the unit's policies are reviewed?' (Maternity Services Advisory Committee, 1984, p. 12)

In the postnatal period,

> each mother should be given such general guidance as she needs on the care and handling of her baby and advice about the professional help she should seek if any aspect of the baby's health care worries her once she has returned home. During the baby's stay in hospital the father should be encouraged to share actively in his care. (Maternity Services Advisory Committee, 1985, p. 5)

This description of postnatal care acknowledges the need for social support, involvement of the woman's partner, health promotion and education as key concepts in postnatal care.

These statements and many others demonstrate the values held by the Committee regarding the need to provide individualised care, continuity of care and to involve the woman and her partner in their care. The documents also demonstrate the Committee's underlying philosophy that birth should take place in hospital. By making these values explicit it is then possible to assess whether these values have been translated into practice or whether they should be modified or changed in the light of new evidence (House of Commons Health Committee, 1992).

Another early statement of philosophy is found in 'The Vision', the document produced by the Association of Radical Midwives (ARM) in 1986 outlining their proposals for the future of maternity services. The document is based on eight principles which demonstrate the philosophy of these midwives:

- That the relationship between mother and midwife is fundamental to good midwifery care.
- That the mother is the central person in the process of care.
- Informed choice in childbirth for women.
- Full utilization of midwives' skills.
- Continuity of care for all childbearing women.
- Community based care.
- Accountability of services to those receiving them.
- Care should do no harm to mother and baby. (Association of Radical Midwives, 1986, p. 2)

These principles have clearly had a widespread effect on midwives and policymakers (House of Commons Health Committee, 1992; Department of Health, 1993a) but it is interesting to speculate how far the 'new feeling' called for in the ARM statement which outlines their philosophy of midwifery practice (citing WHO (1985a) and Flint (1986)) has been generated:

> We wish to change the perception of the general public about midwives so that we can practice the profession of which we have been trained. Midwives are unique in their combination of skill, sensitivity and training, to be 'with women' through one of life's landmark experiences which has long-term effects on the individual, the family and society as a whole. We must generate a new feeling in midwifery. We owe it to ourselves and those we serve. (Association of Radical Midwives, 1986, p. 12)

The values or concepts which are part of the ARM vision and the Maternity Services Association Committee reports are also made explicit in the Royal College of Nursing (1993) document on standards of care for midwifery:

> Midwifery as a profession provides a service to society and possesses a specialist body of knowledge. This knowledge is based on clinical practice supported by relevant research. A profession educates its own practitioners and sets its own standards, adapting the service to meet the changing needs and demands of society and those of the profession.
>
> Each woman is a unique individual with her own beliefs, needs, rights and expectations. This includes the woman's right to negotiate her care and to make an informed choice. Midwifery care should respond to this in order to ensure the delivery of effective individualised care to the woman, her baby and her family. The midwife, through her knowledge, skills and professional expertise, has the responsibility to facilitate this.
>
> Whilst the midwife is the prime care provider, the contribution of others in the health care team is recognised. Co-operation and the mutual recognition of respective roles should enhance the standards of care.
>
> The philosophy also recognises the need to create a safe and supportive environment to provide for the total wellbeing of the woman and her baby. The model of care should encourage autonomy, confidence and self esteem, and contribute towards a satisfying experience of childbirth for the woman and her family. (Royal College of Nursing, 1993, p. 2)

This philosophy includes the following values which relate to midwifery: midwifery is a service; midwifery is based on a body of knowledge; midwifery is responsive to changing demands; midwifery takes place within a context of teamwork. The philosophy also expresses values that relate to the childbearing woman: midwifery recognises the individuality of each woman; midwifery encourages women to be involved in negotiating their care; midwifery is concerned with developing the self-confidence of women. The standard statements that follow on, for example, access to and flexibility of services and woman-centred care, identify structure, process and outcome criteria which may be adopted locally to demonstrate to what extent the philosophy is evident in practice. These criteria can be used to measure the extent to which the concepts, which are made explicit in the philosophy of care, are actually realised in that care. Without this clear statement of concepts it is not possible to assess the extent to which women have choice, can exercise control or experience continuity in care.

At the local level philosophies developed by midwives indicate the extent to which they share the same values or concepts as those stated in national philosophies (above) and international statements (below). In Chapter 7, reference is made to a locally developed model and philosophy (Telfer, 1991 and Carter, 1992) and the philosophy which informs this model is reproduced below:

PHILOSOPHY OF CARE

Midwives are expected to provide midwifery care which will:

Be designed to meet the individual needs of mothers and babies and their families.

Be supported by respect for individual autonomy, dignity, values and beliefs.

Be planned in partnership with the woman and her family.

Empower the woman and her family to make their own choices and decisions about the plan of care.

Consider physical, psychological, social, cultural, spiritual and educational needs.

Be based on appropriate research findings.

Be informed by compassion, commitment, conscience, confidence and competence.

Have a systematic approach to assessment, planning, implementing, recording and evaluating care.

Recognise that pregnancy is a normal physiological process.

Ensure effective communication systems between the midwife and the woman and her family, and with other health care professionals.

Acknowledge the importance of continuity of care by a team of midwives.

Take due consideration of available resources.

Be given by midwives who are encouraged to pursue their personal and professional development and who have complied with the statutory requisites for continuing education.

Be in accordance with local and statutory requirements. (Carter, 1992)

The philosophy adopted by midwives in West Glamorgan Health Authority indicates the extent to which midwives in different parts of the country share the same values and concepts of midwifery:

Pregnancy and birth are normal, physiological events in the lives of the majority of women. The midwife is privileged in that she shares in these experiences, with women and their families. The relationship between mother and midwife is fundamental to good midwifery care.

The mother is at all times the central person in the process of care. She has a right to informed choice and to receive care, which she has chosen from safe and valid alternatives, and in an environment appropriate to her needs.

It is the midwives' responsibility to enable and empower each woman to make informed choices.

Through her clinical expertise and interpersonal skills, the midwife aims to ensure optimum physical and emotional wellbeing during the woman's pregnancy, childbirth and early parenthood.

When complications are anticipated or manifest, the midwife refers to a medical practitioner or appropriate member of the health care team whilst continuing to give care and support. (West Glamorgan Health Authority, 1992, p. 3)

These philosophies include concepts which are also found in the International Code of Ethics for Midwives adopted by the International Confederation of Midwives in 1993 (International Confederation of Midwives, 1993). This code or philosophy 'to guide the education, practice and research of the midwife' (ICM, 1993, p. 169) is based on the concepts of respect of women as persons, justice for all people, equity of access to health care, trust, and the dignity of members of society (ICM, 1993). These concepts are included in the different sections of the code which describe the midwife–woman relationship; the practice of midwifery; midwives' professional responsibilities; and the advancement of midwifery knowledge and practice. The following examples illustrate the concept of respect for persons (which includes respect for colleagues), and the concern of midwives for practices in the wider community:

Midwives respect a woman's informed right of choice and promote the woman's acceptance of responsibility for the outcomes of her choices.

Midwives support and sustain each other in their professional roles, and actively nurture their own and other's sense of selfworth.

Midwives provide care for women and childbearing families with respect for cultural diversity while also working to eliminate harmful practices within those same cultures. (International Confederation of Midwives, 1993, p. 169)

The above code introduces the concept of concern for the health practices of the wider community while the philosophy of the New Zealand College of Midwives also includes the concept of the lifecycle:

Midwifery is a profession concerned with the promotion of women's health. It is centred upon sexuality and reproduction and an understanding of women as healthy individuals progressing through the life cycle.

Midwifery is: dynamic in its approach; based upon an integration of knowledge that is derived from the arts and sciences; tempered by experience and research; collaborative with other health professionals.

Midwifery is holistic by nature, combining an understanding of the social, emotional, cultural, spiritual, psychological and physical ramifications of women's reproductive health experience; actively promoting and protecting women's wellness; promoting health awareness in women's significant others; enhancing the health status of the baby when the pregnancy is on-going.

Midwifery care is delivered in a manner that is flexible, creative, empowering and supportive.

Midwifery care takes place in partnership with women.

Continuity of midwifery care enhances and protects the normal process of childbirth. (New Zealand College of Midwifery, 1992, p. 7)

In New Zealand, midwifery has recently re-emerged as a dynamic force in the provision of maternity care (Abel and Kearns, 1991) and in their logo the New Zealand midwives emphasise the interrelationships between midwives and women in the circular repetition of: 'Midwives Need Women Need Midwives' (New Zealand College of Midwives (Inc), 1992, p. 6). The dynamic nature of midwifery practice in New Zealand is reflected in the above philosophy, the code of ethics and standards of practice formulated by the New Zealand College of Midwives. Again these standards appear to lay more stress on the responsibilities midwives have to the community than do similar statements of philosophy formulated by midwives in Britain.

This brief overview of philosophies underpinning midwifery practice illustrates the strides that midwives have made since the early 1980s in defining the essential elements of midwifery care. Examination of the concepts indicates the consensus that appears to exist between midwives, across cultures, in relation to the fundamental concepts which apply to the care of the childbearing woman and her family. One way to develop theory in midwifery would be to examine such statements as those above, to identify the concepts within the statements, the relationships between the concepts, and to test these relationships through research, thus developing the understanding and theory on which midwifery care is based. This approach to theory development is illustrated in the work of Mercer (1986) and Lehrman (1981) discussed in Chapter 6.

The descriptions of the values held by midwives and the type of practitioner a midwife should or could be illustrate the enormous range of beliefs that midwives hold about their practice. These beliefs can be considered as lying at different points on the continuum of models which lie between the model of pregnancy as a normal life-event and the model of pregnancy as normal only in retrospect, the medical/obstetric model of pregnancy. This continuum will now be discussed in the light of the above description of the range of beliefs and values held by midwives. The consequences these different models have for practice, for action, will also be considered.

PREGNANCY AS A NORMAL LIFE-EVENT VERSUS OBSTETRIC MEDICAL MODEL OF PREGNANCY

The continuum between these models and the main beliefs and consequences for action associated with these models are illustrated in Figure 5.1.

The medical/obstetric model of pregnancy defines pregnancy as a potentially pathological condition requiring medical intervention. This model stresses physical care rather than care of the whole person (Weitz and Sullivan, 1985). Pregnancy is treated as an illness and women are encouraged to view themselves as patients (Comaroff, 1977). The outcomes of care within this model are measured by physical and physiological criteria (Oakley, 1980). As Chalmers *et al.* (1980) comment: 'Clinicians see reproduction as a medical and potentially

Medical model of pregnancy ◄───► Pregnancy as a normal life event

Perspectives	*Perspectives*
1. Normal in retrospect	1. Normal in anticipation
2. The unusual case as interesting	2. Each pregnancy a unique event
3. Prevention of physical complications	3. Development of the individual through experience of pregnancy
4. Doctor in charge	4. Woman and family major decision-makers
5. Information restricted	5. Information shared
Outcomes	*Outcomes*
6. Live, healthy mother and baby	6. Live, healthy mother and baby and satisfaction of individual needs

(Reproduced from Bryar (1985), Diagram 5.3, p. 61)

Figure 5.1   *Continuum contrasting the medical model of pregnancy and the model of pregnancy as a normal life-event*

pathological process, the success of which is to be measured in terms of perinatal mortality rates and guaranteed by the surveillance of professional experts' (Chalmers *et al.*, 1980, p. 844).

This concern with the abnormal has been used to determine the care provided to all women regardless of risk:

the Peel Report provided a major impetus for confinement being in hospital and we do not think this trend should change. Even in low risk cases there is evidence that the risk of developing an abnormality during labour is approximately 10% and we remain convinced that all confinements should take place in hospital. (Royal College of Obstetricians and Gynaecologists, 1982, p. 24, cited by Opoku, 1992, p. 120)

Oakley (1987; 1980) has described the medical/obstetric model as consisting of the following features: the definition of pregnancy as a medical and therefore pathological process about which doctors are the sole experts; the limited definition of the criteria of reproductive success – perinatal and maternal mortality rates; the divorce of reproduction, as an illness, from its social context and the typification of women as by nature maternal.

The alternative model of pregnancy emphasises pregnancy as a normal life-event:

The medical definition of pregnancy is opposed, both within the health services and in wider society, by a cogent view which asserts that pregnancy and childbirth are natural processes; as such they are best managed by the woman herself, with assistance from, rather than control by professional agents. (Comaroff, 1977, p. 115).

Within this model pregnancy is viewed as a natural process and a period of growth (Breen, 1975; Weitz and Sullivan, 1985) in which decision-making is restored to women, preventing the potentially serious consequences of the passive role assigned to women within the medical model (Gaskin, 1977; National Childbirth Trust, 1981; Brackbill *et al.*, 1984). This model of pregnancy puts the woman at the centre, rather than the obstetrician or the midwife. She is the person who is able to make choices and reach decisions about the type of care she would prefer and where she would prefer her baby to be born based on information from, among others, the midwives, doctors and obstetricians who may be involved in her care.

The WHO study *Having a Baby in Europe* (1985a) strongly emphasises the need to attend to what are termed the social aspects of pregnancy:

The hospital birth in Europe today has focused on the biology of birth while forgetting it is equally a social phenomenon. The value of the birth experience in the development of the individual woman and the way in which her development in turn affects her pregnancy, her childbirth and her functioning as a mother, has been forgotten. Part of the development of any individual is learning how to cope with new and/or difficult situations. Coping includes maintaining, as far as humanly possible, an alert conscious control of one's situation. This is why choice is essential if giving birth is to be a positive experience for the woman, since it is the most important means of remaining in control in difficult times. (World Health Organization, 1985a, p. 97).

Early in this report the startling statement is made that in Europe 'it is no longer known what normal (i.e. "non-medicalised") birth is' (WHO, 1985a, p. 1), which indicates that the medical/obstetric model pervades the care of the childbearing woman throughout Europe.

Opoku (1992) identifies two uses of the term normal in the literature. The first uses the word to mean common and 'includes common procedures such as episiotomy, artificial rupture of membranes, intravenous infusions and electronic foetal monitoring' (Opoku, 1992, p. 121). The second use of the term normal is in the sense of natural, birth without intervention. In the continuum above, the model of pregnancy as a normal life-event, however, encompasses something more than these essentially medical definitions: the growth and development of the individual woman.

Currell (1990) considers that there is a need to put the focus on the woman (rather than the health professional). Childbirth is then seen as a process which is a part of the wider life processes experienced by the woman. Childbirth is then seen as a time of great opportunity for growth but equally a time of great potential harm and restrictions on growth. Midwives and obstetricians are therefore in a crucial position to either assist or to inhibit the woman, and potentially her child, to grow. Nurse-midwives in the USA have identified this change in roles and personal growth as the focus of their models of attainment of the maternal role (see Chapter 6; Rubin, 1984; Mercer, 1986).

The medical/obstetric and pregnancy as normal life-event models have been presented at the opposite ends of a continuum. The question then is: what is the model that midwives hold or, what are the models that midwives hold? Opoku (1992) describes the use of the 'normal' pregnancy model by midwives in their efforts to resist medical interventions and to take charge of twin or breech births. This use of the model, as a tool to oppose the power of another profession, is similar to the use of bonding to achieve change in the care of mothers and babies in hospital (see Chapter 4). However, in the 1970s and early 1980s studies showed that midwives aligned themselves with an obstetric model of pregnancy. The majority of midwives work in hospitals in which the care of women as patients has been described (Thomson, 1980; Kirkham, 1983; 1989). Comaroff (1977) observed that midwives demonstrated in their practice adherence to an obstetric model:

> This paradigm was expressed at a number of levels: in explicit reference to the management of women as 'patients'; in the exclusion of non-medical aspects of childbirth from communications with them, in their encouragement of reliance upon medical control over labour; in a reluctance to demystify technical knowledge for the women with whom they dealt. (Comaroff, 1977, p. 126).

Midwives were observed by Kirkham (1983) to give limited information to women, thus limiting their potential for making decisions. Laryea (1980) found that women postnatally emphasised their need for emotional support and teaching while the midwives emphasised physical care, utilising a medical model of pregnancy. The women were reluctant to express their views to midwives, whom they considered did not understand how they felt. In a study of antenatal care, Methven

(1982; 1989) concluded that midwives operated within a medical model of pregnancy and commented that there was a need for midwives to realise the limitations of the medical/obstetric model for care and for expression of their own role. Further evidence of the medical model held by midwives is provided in a study of the introduction of individualised care in a maternity unit. The midwives were involved in the construction of a combined assessment schedule to be used in care of the childbearing woman. This assessment schedule contained 134 items, the majority of which indicate an obstetric/physical focus of care, under 20 items indicating a wider view of pregnancy as a time of social change, a time for education and personal growth (Bryar, 1985).

The flexibility of the term 'normal' highlighted by Opoku (1992) means that this term can be used to cover a type of care that includes a great deal of professional control:

> The 'normal' model is not against home births supported by adequate backup for emergencies and it favours 'low-tech' births in consultant or GP units. (Opoku, 1992, p. 121)

Arney (1982) argues that the type of control described by Opoku (a midwife) is a feature of the hidden control built into alternative forms of care. The great fear for obstetricians, Arney (1982) suggests, is not the case which has been mishandled and ends in tragedy but the woman who has her baby outside of and unknown by the system of obstetrical care. He describes the alternative birth centres and places such as the Farm in Tennessee (Gaskin, 1977) as providing alternative care but within obstetric control. These alternatives have been developed within the obstetric rule (medical model) which maintains safety as the most important factor. Through provision of such alternatives, Arney (1982) argues that the woman becomes responsible for her safety (for maintenance of the obstetric rule), making it even harder for her to opt out of the care system:

> Alternatives to birth have arisen not in opposition to the rule that birth should occur within a flexible system of obstetrical alternatives in which a woman's experience can gain prominence against a background of obstetrical expertise and safety; alternatives have arisen *within* this rule. The rule informs and facilitates alternatives, and the rule, in turn, is strengthened by their existence as they push the apparent limitations imposed by the rule further and further outward. The rule comes to resemble a liberating rather than constraining force....The world of imagined possibilities comes to be defined in terms of the options available under the rule. The 'flexible systems'

rule constrains imagination and becomes the force that holds together the panoptic machine that controls birth. (Arney, 1982, p. 240)

DeVries (1993) argues that midwives have lost power and are in danger as a profession, as they have defined their area of practice as the normal, as low-risk. He argues that professional power is associated with emphasising risk. However, Welford (1993), in a discussion of birthing rooms, suggests that this definition of low risk may in fact increase midwifery power. Through the definition of low-risk, obstetricians are excluded from care but that care, such as that provided in birthing rooms by midwives, takes place within the confines of the hospital, reducing obstetric concern (Arney, 1982). Welford (1993) suggests that the establishment of birthing rooms may in fact reduce women's choice and prevent the establishment of truly radical services:

> I would argue that the birthing room as we know it is actually a compromise between truly radical changes that might allow the birthplace to empower women and midwives and what more traditional colleagues feel comfortable with. (Welford, 1993, p. 35)

The analysis by Arney (1982) and Welford (1993) may be painful for midwives but they need to be considered, as efforts are made to identify midwifery models of care. These authors indicate the need to examine each value carefully and thoroughly for its true meaning and the consequences it has for practice.

The midwife, according to some authors, appears to hold a medical/obstetric model of pregnancy and this model may, in some cases, be reinforced by the setting within which they work. The adoption of the medical model may have benefits for the midwife at the individual and professional levels. The presentation by the midwife of a stereotyped image may prevent 'patients' discussing threatening topics with the midwife (Jourard, 1971; Comaroff, 1977). The alternative model may lead to the discussion of such topics as the woman's emotional needs or psycho-social aspects of pregnancy that the midwife may not feel prepared (either emotionally or professionally) to discuss (Breen, 1975; Laryea, 1980; see Chapter 2).

The organisation in which the midwife is working, and the organisational role relationships in that organisation (see Figures 3.1 and 3.2), may also have a significant impact on the type of care that the midwife is able to provide (see Chapter 3) and the models of care held by midwives. Weitz and Sullivan (1985), for example, found that lay midwives who held a model of pregnancy which was focused on women adopted aspects of the medical model following licensure. This suggests that while licensure is to be welcomed – for example, most recently in Canada – it may have unexpected consequences for the care that the midwives provide.

A study of nurses in an Australian hospital showed that the nurses identified with other health professionals to such a great extent that this was actually to the detriment of the patients. For example, nurses went out of their way to prevent the doctor being 'put down' in front of patients. In one example given by a nurse, a doctor was having difficulty inserting a cannula. This nurse said that she could give the doctor a hint that he was distressing the patient. But even though she commented: 'The patient would be crying, you know, and he'd just keep on trying. It was terrible; it's a shame someone didn't grab him and show him' (Buckenham and McGrath, 1983, p. 57), this nurse had such a strong sense of responsibility to the health team and to her 'superordinate team-mate'(p. 57) that she did not intervene. The needs of the doctors came before the needs of the patients and the position of the nurses as part of the professional health team was maintained. This was more important to these nurses than the very painful role they would have had to adopt in relation to their other colleagues if they were going to take patient care, and the patient advocacy that goes with it, as their central focus (Buckenham and McGrath, 1983). The description of the political and other constraints on the practice of midwifery provided by Garcia *et al.* (1990) suggests that these experiences found in a nursing setting may not be unique but may also affect the practice of midwifery.

Summary

In this chapter the aim has been to demonstrate the concepts that midwives hold which may be found in their writings about midwifery care. In most cases the concepts identified have been implicit rather than explicit in the literature. Statements of philosophies of midwifery care provide a more explicit description of these concepts. There is a vast body of midwifery literature, a small part of which has been considered here. This review does indicate, however, that the concepts and models of midwifery practice may have undergone considerable change since the early 1980s. This raises questions as to the extent to which these new models are evident in practice.

The chapter ended with a discussion of the medical model approach to childbearing and the approach based on the view of pregnancy as a normal life-event. Organisational and professional limitations on practice within the second model which may in subtle ways support the medical model of childbearing were considered. Adherence to either the medical/obstetric model or to the model of pregnancy as a normal life-event or to a model that lies in between these extremes, it was suggested, has consequences for both the childbearing woman and the midwife.

Activities

Having read this chapter it is suggested that you undertake the following activities to assist you in identification of the concepts which inform your own practice.

1 With reference to the books discussed in the first part of this chapter identify the concepts which the authors suggest should form the basis of midwifery practice.
2 Examine in detail one midwifery textbook and identify the model of midwifery practice on which it is based and identify the concepts that make up that model.
3 Examine the midwifery philosophy which has been developed in your place of work. What are the concepts contained in this philosophy? What are the measurable indicators or criteria which you could use to examine whether this philosophy is being put into practice?
4 Are the concepts, identified in Activity 3 above, the same as those you identified in your own philosophy of midwifery practice in Chapter 2? If not, what consequences does this difference in the concepts you hold and those in the local philosophy have for your practice?
5 What assumptions does the medical/obstetric model make about women and childbirth? How does the model affect the assessment information that is collected by the midwife? How does the model influence the participation of the woman in her own care?
6 Consider the arguments put forward by Arney (1982) and Welford (1993). What choices do women have in relation to place of birth, where you are working? How are these choices constrained?
7 What assumptions does the model of pregnancy as a normal life-event make about women and childbirth? How does the model affect the assessment information that is collected by the midwife? How does the model influence the participation of the woman in her own care?
8 Consider your own practice and identify any instances where the needs of other health care practitioners came before the needs of the childbearing woman. What factors contributed to your behaving in this way? What action could you take to ensure that in similar circumstances in the future the needs of the childbearing woman might be more adequately met?

CHAPTER SIX

Five midwifery theorists

The reader is assured of the investigator's belief in the credibility of alternative approaches, and offers the challenge of multiple models of nurse-midwifery practice. Of greatest importance is the continued evolution of nurse-midwifery through scientific research. (Lehrman, 1988, p. 119)

INTRODUCTION

It is evident from Chapter 5 that midwives hold a large number of concepts and a range of mental pictures about their practice. Chapter 5 illustrates one approach to theory development, the description by midwives of the elements that underpin their practice. These descriptions may then be discussed, revised and adapted by others, but their clear articulation allows discussion to take place. This chapter continues the exploration of the individual's definition of the situation (see Figure 3.1) which was started in Chapter 5.

In this chapter the work of four nurse-midwives and a midwife who have explicitly sought to identify the theory underlying midwifery practice is described. These nurse-midwives and midwife have considered the models and theory underpinning practice and have then, in all cases bar one (Wiedenbach), gone on to test the concepts making up the theory or model through research.

It is often argued that there has been no theory development in midwifery. The preceding chapter has shown that the explanation of concepts underpinning practice has always been an implicit aim of midwife educators or leaders but this chapter shows that explicit research on developing midwifery theory has been taking place since the 1960s.

REVA RUBIN: ATTAINMENT OF THE MATERNAL ROLE

Rubin is a nurse-midwife whose research and theory development has had a wide influence on the care of childbearing women and research and theorising about that care in the USA. Her research stemmed from research questions stimulated by role theory and was aimed at exploring the development of the maternal role. This, then, is an example of deductive research: questions were raised in the investigator's mind by role theory, and research was then undertaken to collect data to provide information about the stages and activities involved in the attainment of the maternal role. In this way, inductive reasoning (from the data) was combined with deductive reasoning (from established theory) to develop a theory of maternal role attainment (see Chapter 2).

Rubin (1967a and 1967b) describes the theoretical issues on which her research was based, which are concerned with role and performance of roles. A distinction is made between the concept of position which is described as the social status assigned to someone (for example, teacher or mother), and the concept of role, which is described as the activities and actions carried out by the individual demonstrating occupancy of a certain position. Individuals hold different positions at different stages of their lives and hold a number of positions at one time – for example, daughter, mother, friend. 'Actions, organised around positions, comprise roles' (Rubin, 1967a, p. 237).

Roles are acquired through a process of learning which is achieved through a series of activities. Rubin's work is aimed at identifying how women take on the role of mother (maternal role) and thus (by implication) what interventions or actions might assist or have a negative effect on this process.

The theoretical basis for her study is given in much greater depth in *Maternal Identity and the Maternal Experience* (Rubin, 1984) but the essential question addressed by the research over a considerable number of years is as follows:

> The problem studied and reported here was how a particular adult role is acquired, specifically the maternal role. What are the processes involved in the acquisition of the maternal role? Who are the models or referrants for maternal role expectations? (Rubin, 1967a, pp. 237–8)

In the initial study, data were collected by a number of graduate students, as they undertook care of women in antenatal clinics and postnatal settings, through interviews and telephone conversations. The data from these interactions were recorded by the students, following the interaction, which might have lasted from one to four hours (clearly there are methodological questions which may be asked about such a method of data collection). The data relating to the problems of becoming a mother were then coded and analysed. From this analysis Rubin identified four tasks that a woman has to complete to achieve the maternal role identity. This analysis was supplemented and modified over the next 20 years with observations of over 6000 women.

Rubin's research and writing covers a period of more than a quarter of century, during which her terminology changed. The following description of the four tasks of pregnancy is taken from Rubin (1984):

> The objectives of the woman's efforts during pregnancy are: a) to ensure safe passage of herself and the baby during pregnancy and childbirth, b) to ensure social acceptance for herself and her child, c) to increase the affinial ties in the construction of the image and identity of the 'I' and 'you' and d) to explore in depth the meaning of the transitive act of giving/receiving (Rubin, 1984, p. 10).

These tasks or goals of activity during pregnancy and the puerperium are described more succinctly by Josten (1981) as:

1. ensuring physical wellbeing of herself and the baby;
2. social acceptance of herself and her child by people who are significant to them both;
3. attachment to the baby;
4. understanding of the complexities of mothering.

From the data Rubin (1967a) identified three aspects of the maternal role identity: 'the ideal image, the self image and the body image' (p. 240).

The ideal image comprises all the ideas that the woman had about the positive attributes and activities of women who are mothers. The self image comprises the attributes that the woman saw herself as possessing from her experience: 'Self image was used as the representation of the consistent "myself"...' (Rubin, 1967a, p. 240). The body image is related to changes in the body during pregnancy and the significance of those changes in terms of the progress of the pregnancy.

The maternal identity is achieved by a process of taking-in activities, taking-on activities and letting-go activities. In 1967 Rubin described five operations or means by which the maternal identity is incorporated into the woman's image of herself:

> Taking-on activities: mimicry and role play
> Taking-in activities: fantasy and introjection–projection–rejection
> Letting-go activities: grief-work

By 1984 mimicry and role play are defined together as Replication; fantasy remains as a separate operation, but incorporates grief-work; and introjection–projection–rejection becomes dedifferentiation (Rubin, 1984).

Mimicry involves the replication of actions and behaviours carried out by role-models (for example, other women who are or have been pregnant) and learning from a variety of sources about events in the future: what the delivery will be like, how the baby will be in the first few days:

> The environment is searched for models (Rubin, 1967a). Suddenly the world seems filled with women who are or have been in some situation of childbearing, a factor not so much of serendipity as of selective searching. Newspaper items, magazine articles, books, television programmes, the grocery and shopping mall, the waiting room and coffee shop near the doctor's office, as well as reminiscent anecdotes in family and social group gatherings add to the same population. Both the favourable and unfavourable experiences become situation-specific models for adoption, if favourable, for avoidance if unfavourable. (Rubin, 1984, p. 40)

In role play, women act out roles that they will be undertaking in the future. For example, they babysit for friends' children, undertake feeding or child care activities. This role-play may be something that actually takes place or something that takes place in the imagination.

Replication (taking-on activities) assists the woman, according to the model proposed by Rubin, to understand how someone who is pregnant, or a new mother, behaves. Fantasy and the other operations of the taking-in phase enable the woman to develop an understanding of how she will behave.

In fantasy the woman imagines the future for herself. For example, what the birth will be like, what the baby will wear and the future relationships with other members of the family.

In grief-work the woman reviews her past roles and relinquishes those roles which are no longer appropriate or possible; letting-go takes place:

> Grief-work is a review, in memory, of the attachments and associated events of a former self (role). The experiences, interpersonal and situational, associated with the former self include the actual and the hoped for, the pleasant and unpleasant. The review in the memory of the details of the former-self serve to loosen the ties with the former-self. (Rubin, 1967a, pp. 243–4)

Introjection–projection–rejection is an active process in which the woman compares the available models with her view of herself and makes active decisions about adopting or rejecting particular models. This activity is differentiated from mimicry in which an activity, such as wearing maternity clothes, is copied. For example, mimicry may occur postnatally when a woman copies (or is made to follow in some

instances) the bathing 'procedure' with her baby but introjection–
projection–rejection has occurred when, at home, she develops her own
approach to bathing based on what she has learnt in hospital and
elsewhere.

> Introjection–projection–rejection was the sum and substance of the
> bulk of the apparently casual woman-talk. It included clothing,
> cooking, walking, talking, childrearing, childbearing and personal re-
> lationships. It was the substance and essence, in detail, of what was
> involved in becoming or being a woman and particularly in becom-
> ing or being a mother. (Rubin, 1967a, p. 243)

The maternal role identity described in this model comprises the
achievement of the four tasks of pregnancy which are accomplished by
undertaking the operations or activities of mimicry, role play and so
on. Rubin (1967a and 1967b) suggests that this model can be imagined
as a sphere, with the maternal role identity at the centre, surrounded by
the operations. The operations of taking-on (mimicry and role play)
precede the operations of taking-in and letting-go and are thus depicted
as the outer rings of the model as shown in Figure 6.1.

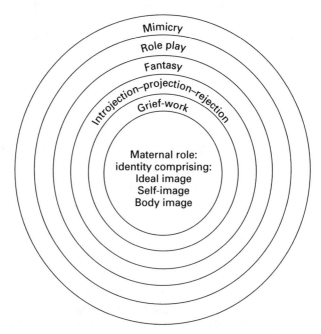

Figure 6.1   *Rubin's model of attainment of the maternal role*

The model may also be presented in a linear fashion as shown in Figure 6.2

Rubin's model will now be considered in relation to the key concepts of person, health, environment and midwifery which were discussed in Chapter 2 as four of the central concepts underpinning midwifery care. The model puts greater emphasis on the person and environment than on health and midwifery.

Person   The model developed by Rubin from integration of theory with vast quantities of empirical data has as its focus the person: the woman and the development of the woman and her identity as a woman, mother and member of society who is a mother – the central concern of the model is with the achievement by the woman of a positive identity as a mother. The achievement of this role can be assessed in terms of attainment of the four tasks of pregnancy. For example, whether the woman has been able to ensure safety for herself and her baby can be assessed in terms of physical outcomes, the health of the baby and the woman. Whether the woman has managed to integrate the baby into her social situation may be assessed in terms of their support systems, financial situation or accommodation.

Health   One of the tasks of pregnancy identified is the maintenance of safety of the woman and baby, including maintenance of health. The maternal identity is described as comprising ideal, self and body images. Throughout pregnancy the body is seen as being of central concern so that health and perceptions of health are particularly important during a time when body changes may be alarming or may not have been experienced before.

Environment   The environment, or social system, is the second major focus of this model. Rubin essentially views maternal behaviour as a social activity which is demonstrated in interactions and relationships with others in the woman's social system. Again, the extent to which the woman has achieved the tasks of pregnancy can be assessed in terms of her relationship with the baby, family, friends, colleagues and health professionals.

Midwifery   This model describes the woman as being involved in an active process of growth and development during pregnancy. During this time she is actively seeking out role-models in the form of people and individuals and integrating these role-models into her picture, or image, of herself. The woman is the central actor in this process. The aim of the midwife, within this model, is to provide interventions which support the operations and achievement of the maternal tasks. For

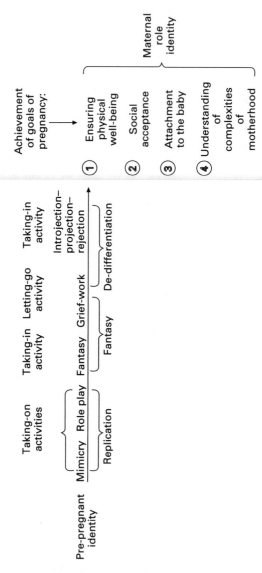

Figure 6.2   Linear representation of Rubin's model of attainment of the maternal role

example, by providing information about food and exercise early in pregnancy the midwife provides a model for the woman to mimic. By providing information about different options for delivery, she provides information which the woman can use in introjection–projection– rejection, and in undertaking observations in labour the midwife helps the woman achieve a safe outcome.

This model places the focus clearly on achievement by the woman of a new role and can be classified with nursing models which are developmental in their focus, although the basis of Rubin's model is in symbolic interactionism. Rubin's model demonstrates the fact that models may draw on a range of different traditions, or paradigms, rather than being based on only one (see Chapter 2). The model helps to identify factors which indicate the health of the woman (in the terms of the model) in its widest sense. Those indicators may be measured during pregnancy to demonstrate to what extent the tasks have been achieved (Josten, 1981) or, at the end of the midwife's care, to provide a summative evaluation of care and achievement of the maternal role identity. The model can be operationalised to provide a basis for practice, a basis on which to audit practice and means of generating research questions.

Use of this model in practice is shown in the Prenatal Assessment Guide described by Josten (1981). This guide was developed to help identify women who might neglect or abuse their babies. The guide consists of a series of indicators associated with the four tasks of pregnancy and includes sample questions to assess whether the tasks are being achieved. The following is an example taken from the guide:

III. Acceptance of child by significant others.

A. Acknowledges acceptance by significant others of the new responsibility inherent in child.

Positive:

2. Partner accepts new responsibility inherent with child.
3. Timely sharing of experience of pregnancy with significant others.

Associated Sample Questions:

1. How does your partner feel about pregnancy?
2. How do your parents feel?
5. What do you think he will be like as a father?
8. Have you and your partner talked about how the baby might change your lives? (Josten, 1981, p. 115).

This guide was used in association with another, which is focused more on child abuse and neglect throughout pregnancy. Together, it is reported in the article, the guides predicted the type of care the woman would give her baby in 87 per cent of cases. Alongside the guide the women were offered support and intervention activities when it was identified that they needed help in achieving the tasks of pregnancy.

Cranley (1981), in a study of maternal–fetal attachment during pregnancy, provides an illustration of the need to test the relationships between concepts in all parts of a model. In this study, the concept of maternal–fetal attachment during pregnancy is tested. A measurement tool was developed which women completed both during pregnancy and in the early postnatal period. This tool measures six aspects of attachment including interaction measured by items on the scale, including: 'I poke the baby to get him/her to poke back.' (Cranley, 1981, p. 282), giving of self, and nesting. The results provided support for the activity of maternal–fetal attachment during pregnancy.

Parts of the model have also been used postnatally; indeed, Martell and Mitchell (1984) cite nine maternity textbooks that base postnatal care on the taking-in and taking-hold phases. In her later work Rubin (1984) describes these processes as taking place throughout pregnancy (as described above: see Figure 6.2) but in 1961 Rubin described, again from observation, taking-in and taking-hold occurring in the immediate postnatal period. Taking-in, where the woman was focused on herself and the immediate past of the labour dominated in the first three days, and taking-hold, where the woman was more orientated to others and to becoming more independent, dominated in days 3–10.

Martell and Mitchell (1984) and Ament (1989) describe studies in which they collected data to assess the extent to which taking-in and taking-hold activities occurred. Ament (1989) found that women did display taking-in and taking-hold behaviours but that taking-in only predominated on day 1 with taking-hold activities predominating from day 2. Martell and Mitchell (1984), on the other hand, found no support for a taking-in phase but did find support for a taking-hold phase that peaked on the second day.

These studies demonstrate the need to test the findings of observational studies in other settings as well as the need to test theoretical propositions. These authors discuss the cultural and organisational changes that have taken place in labour and postnatal care since the 1960s which could also have had a significant effect on the demonstration of these phases as, for example, postnatal hospital stay has been reduced.

Rubin has developed a model of Maternal Role Attainment through a process of deductive reasoning combined with extensive observational research over more than a quarter of a century. While some of the language of the model and descriptions of maternal attributes may be culturally specific, the model provides a picture of the process by which women become mothers and it offers a framework to guide midwifery care in assisting women to attain this role.

RAMONA T. MERCER: THEORIES OF ANTEPARTUM STRESS AND MATERNAL ROLE ATTAINMENT

Mercer is the only theorist whose work has been exclusively concerned with understanding the process of childbearing who is included in a collection considering the work of the major theorists in nursing (Marriner-Tomey, 1989). Bee and Oetting (1989) provide a description of Mercer's distinguished academic career which has spanned over 30 years. During that time her work has been focused on theory-building, research and practice applications of research findings in the field of maternity care. Her work has been greatly influenced by Rubin, who was the professor in maternity nursing at the university where Mercer obtained her doctoral degree. By 1988 Mercer had published four books, over 55 articles, book chapters and reports: a body of work which in itself shows that there has been considerable theory development by nurse-midwives in the care of the childbearing family.

In addition, Mercer has been responsible for the development of a range of measurement tools for use in research which have been widely used by other researchers (see, for example, Fawcett *et al.*, 1993, for use of the Perception of Birth Scale; Marut and Mercer, 1979). Mercer has also been concerned to apply the findings of her research and theory building to practice: 'The concepts theorized by Mercer have been used by nursing in multiple obstetric textbooks. She is often cited as taking the work by Rubin and expanding its utilization. Her theory is extremely practice orientated.' (Bee and Oetting, 1989, p. 299). This concern with the utilisation of theory is shown in the discussion of implications for nursing intervention in *First-Time Motherhood* (Mercer, 1986) and in articles such as 'The Nurse and Maternal Tasks of the Early Postpartum' (Mercer, 1981a). For example, in this article, Mercer comments on the tasks that the woman has to undertake in the early postnatal days and indicates that these tasks 'encompass far more than "bonding" to her infant' (Mercer, 1981a, p. 344). One of the tasks that has been identified theoretically and confirmed through research observation is the task of integrating the labour and birth experiences. Ways in which the nurse/midwife may assist the woman in this task are suggested:

> When the nurse asks, 'What was your labor and delivery like?' this requires creative listening to hear what the woman is really saying when she answers. One way to facilitate the work of fitting in the 'missing pieces' and integrating the birth is through a review of the labor and delivery with the nurse who was with her. (Mercer, 1981a, p. 344)

Another interesting feature of Mercer's work, which is noted by Bee and Oetting (1989) and applies also to many of the nurse theorists, is that it has been utilised by a large number of graduate students who were supervised by Mercer. Such a programme of ongoing research provides further evidence of the utility of the theory or provides information which can lead to modification of a theory.

Through all her work, Mercer demonstrates the integration of deductive theory building, from the literature and other theory, with inductive theory building from observation in practice. This is shown, for example, in an article which describes the construction of three models which help in the study of antenatal stress on families (Mercer, 1986), discussed below. Her work is concerned with the testing of the models through research and the systematic collection of data to test the relationships suggested by the evidence on which the models are based.

Mercer has undertaken theory building and research in two main areas: the effects of antepartum stress and attainment of the maternal role.

The effect of antepartum stress on the family

In British literature on antenatal care there is a concern to provide support during pregnancy to reduce the effects of poor social circumstances, lack of social support and poor self-esteem among women (Chalmers *et al.*, 1981). The introduction to a report on the Newcastle Community Midwifery Care Project (Davies and Evans, 1981) and other research indicate that this concern has been linked to poor perinatal outcomes (Oakley *et al.*, 1990). The evaluation of the Newcastle study considered the effects of the project on continuity of care; labour and delivery outcomes and postnatal outcomes, including rates of admission to the special-care baby unit and choices about feeding and rates of breast-feeding. Mercer's research is concerned with a number of other measures of the effects of antenatal stress relating to the functioning of the family unit. Mercer and her colleagues have been seeking to understand the effects of antenatal stress on family functioning, as a whole; on functioning of pairs of individuals in a family, and on health status.

Mercer *et al.* (1986) identify six variables from research and other literature which are related to health status, dyadic relationships and family functioning: antepartum stress, social support, self-esteem, sense of mastery, anxiety and depression. The outcome variables (or dependent variables) are defined as follows.

For health status they were: 'the mother's and father's perception of their prior health, current health, health outlook, resistance-susceptibility to illness, health worry concerns, sickness orientation, and rejection of the sick role'(Mercer *et al.*, 1986, p. 342). Infant health status is defined as the extent of any pathology combined with the parental rating of the infant's overall health.

Antepartum stress is described as resulting from a combination of negative life-events and the level of risk associated with the pregnancy: '*Antepartum stress* is defined as a complication of pregnancy or at-risk condition (pregnancy risk) and negatively perceived life events' (Mercer *et al.*, 1986, p. 339).

'The *family* is defined as a dynamic system which includes subsystems – individuals (mother, father, fetus/infant) and dyads (mother–father, mother–fetus/infant, and father–fetus/infant) within the overall family system.' (Mercer *et al.*, 1986, p. 339)

Each of the independent variables, for example, social support and self-esteem, is defined and the theoretical basis for each variable discussed. Three models are then presented which suggest the relationships between the independent variables and the dependent variables of health status (of the individual), dyadic relationships and family functioning. These models consider antenatal stress in relation to: (i) the individual; (ii) the dyads; (iii) family functioning.

The family is described as a large system embracing sub-systems, the dyads of mother–father, mother–fetus/infant and others. As we have seen earlier (Chapter 3), systems are subject to influence from the outside and similarly Mercer *et al.* (1986) describe the outcomes (actions, in terms of family functioning or health status) as being affected by external influences. These include the whole spectrum of negative life-events. But Mercer *et al.* (1986) make the point that the effects of negative life-events and pregnancy risk may be ameliorated (or accentuated) by the individual characteristics of those who make up the family and by the social support that is available.

In a later article, Mercer *et al.* (1988) present the results of a study which was undertaken to test one of the three models of antepartum stress. This study considered the effects of antepartum stress on family functioning (the third outcome area mentioned above). Within the model it is suggested that variables have either negative or positive effects on family functioning as indicated in this description of the model:

> Stress from negative life-events and pregnancy risk were predicted to have direct negative effects on self-esteem and health status; self-esteem, health status, and social support were predicted to have direct positive effects on sense of mastery; sense of mastery was predicted to have direct negative effects on anxiety and depression which in turn have direct negative effects on family functioning. (Mercer *et al.*, 1988, p. 269)

These relationships are shown in Figure 6.3. The relationships in the model were tested in a study of women who had been admitted to hospital with high-risk pregnancies. These women were compared with a group of women who had low-risk pregnancies. In addition, the partners of half the women in both groups were also interviewed. Mercer *et al.* (1988) make the point that much research on pregnancy has been from the woman's viewpoint and that there is a need to consider family functioning from the viewpoint of the male partner as well. Data was collected in relation to each of the six independent variables (self-esteem, social support and the others) using a variety of data-collection tools, including an index of general health and measures of social support. The dependent variable, family functioning, was measured using a family-functioning measurement instrument. The data was collected when the women were between 24 and 34 weeks pregnant.

The data were then analysed using a range of statistical tests to test the study hypotheses:

Hypotheses

I. High-risk women experiencing antenatal hospitalization and their partners will report less optimal family functioning than low-risk women and their partners.

II. Expectant partners will report similar levels of family functioning. (Mercer *et al.*, 1988, p. 269)

The study findings supported the first hypothesis but did not support the second hypothesis in relation to the partners of the low-risk women. Using statistical tests, the researchers are able to show the impact of each of the variables on family functioning and to show the different predictive values of the different variables for women in the low-risk group and the high risk-group. This enabled the

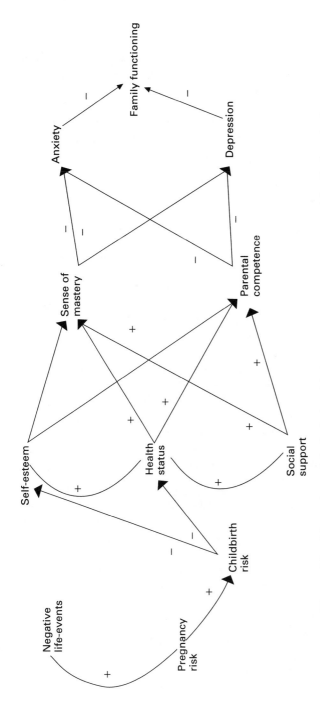

Figure 6.3   *Mercer's model of relationship between antepartum stress and family functioning*

researchers to redraw their model of the effect of antepartum stress on family functioning. Two different models emerge from the data, one which demonstrates the relationship of the variables in the case of the low-risk women and the other which does the same for the high-risk women. These models may now be further tested and modified. This information, derived from testing a model, regarding the variables which are of particular importance in predicting the experience of antenatal stress and the effects of that stress on family functioning, may be utilised in practice in determining priority areas for action by midwives.

Maternal role attainment

The underlying concern in Mercer's work is with attainment of the maternal role: 'Becoming a mother means taking on a new identity. Taking on a new identity involves a complete rethinking and redefining of self' (Mercer, 1986, p. 3). The reason for the interest of American nurse-midwives in attainment of the maternal role may appear to be self-evident but Mercer indicates that interest in the role is important because some women have difficulty taking on the maternal role which, Mercer suggests, has consequences for their children: 'While most women achieve the role successfully, approximately one to two million mothers [in the USA] experience difficulty with the role, as evidenced by the number of abused or neglected children'(Mercer, 1981b).

Mercer (as does Rubin), takes an interactionist approach to understanding the process by which people take on new roles. The interactionist view is that the way an individual takes on and acts out a particular role is dependent on the reactions and interactions that they have with people in their environment, for example, their partner, the infant, their family and other people:

> Maternal role attainment is an interactional and developmental process occurring over a period of time, during which the mother becomes attached to her infant, acquires competence in the caretaking tasks involved in the role, and expresses pleasure and gratification in the role. Role-taking involves the active interaction of the role-taker and the role partner; each responds to cues from the other and alters behaviour according to the other's response. (Mercer, 1986, p. 24)

The expression of a role by an individual will also be affected by their past experiences and view of themselves (Mercer, 1981b, 1986; Dunnington and Glazer, 1991). Mercer (1981b) describes the theoretical base of her research in role acquisition theory, which identifies four stages to role acquisition: anticipatory, formal, informal and personal stages:

> The anticipatory stage is the period prior to incumbency when an individual begins social and psychological adjustment to the role by learning the expectations of the role. The formal stage begins with actual incumbency during which role behaviours are largely guided by formal, consensual expectations of others in the individual's social system. The informal stage begins as the individual develops unique ways of dealing with the role that are not conveyed by the social system. During the final, or personal, stage of role acquisition, an individual imposes an individual style on the role performance, and others largely accept the enactment. Social adjustment has occurred through role modification, and psychological adjustment has resulted in the individual's feeling a congruence of self and role. (Mercer, 1981b, p. 74)

While Rubin describes many of the activities associated with taking on the maternal role as occurring in pregnancy and up to six months after the birth of the child (Mercer, 1981b), Mercer's theoretical model indicates that the majority of the role-taking activities occur after the birth of the child, and that attainment of the maternal role may occur between three and ten months after the birth. Mercer has identified eleven independent variables which influence the attainment of the maternal role (the dependent variable) and a number of confounding variables. Confounding variables include the woman's cultural background, which will have an effect on the way she perceives the maternal role and the way that she adopts the role. Confounding variables affect both the independent and dependent variables.

Mercer has undertaken extensive research describing the relationship between these variables and attainment of the maternal role. These variables can be grouped into maternal, infant and other/confounding variables.

Maternal variables
1 Maternal age at first birth
2 Perceptions of the birth experience
3 Early maternal–infant separation
4 Social stress
5 Social support
6 Self-concept
7 Personality traits
8 Child-rearing attitudes
9 Maternal health status

Infant variables
1 Temperament
2 Infant health

Other/confounding variables
1 Ethnic background
2 Marital status
3 Socioeconomic status

An interesting aspect of Mercer's work is the stress that she places on the effect of the infant and the infant's personality on the taking of the maternal role by the mother. Each of the above variables is discussed by Mercer (1981b; 1986) and the theoretical base and research evidence for each variable are presented. Taking social support as an example, Mercer refers to research which identifies four types of support: emotional, informational, physical and appraisal which she defines as follows:

> *Emotional support* is defined as feeling loved, cared for, trusted, and understood. *Informational support* helps the individual to help herself by providing information that is useful in dealing with the problem and/or situation. *Physical support* is a direct type of help, such as baby-sitting, lending money, etc. *Appraisal support* is information that tells the role-taker how she is performing in the role; it enables the individual to evaluate herself in relationship to others' performance in the role. (Mercer, 1986, p. 14)

Mercer (1986) goes on to describe research evidence of the existence and need for different types of support in pregnancy, postnatally, by fathers and in general.

The influence of these variables has been investigated by Mercer in a longitudinal study of 242 women aged 15 to 42 years (Mercer, 1986). The main aim of this research was to identify whether age had any effect on attainment of the maternal role. Secondary aims were to identify the effect of the other variables, either individually or in combination, on the maternal role and to identify from the data collected whether there were any other factors which appeared to affect the maternal role (Mercer, 1981b; 1986). The study involved the collection of data using a battery of measurement tools from the sample on five different occasions, from the early postnatal period through to the end of the first year.

The findings from this study are extensive and are presented in relation to three age-groups of women: aged 15–19, 20–29 and 30–42. One of the main conclusions that is reached is that maternal age 'was not a predictor of maternal role attainment when, race, educational level, and marital status were controlled' (Mercer, 1986, p. 320). The younger mothers were, however, handicapped by their low incomes and poor self-concept, but Mercer makes the point that almost half of the women in this age-group dropped out of the study. Relationships were found between age and other variables measured which indicates that age is an important variable in any model constructed to understand the attainment of the maternal role.

The findings include a large amount of statistical information and also extensive excerpts from the interviews with the women during the first year. Mercer (1986) uses the data to present a model of adaptation to the maternal role in the first year which combines four phases of adaptation at three levels. The four phases described are:

> ...*physical recovery phase*, from birth to 1 month; an *achievement phase*, from 2 to 4 or 5 months; a *disruption phase*, from 6 to 8 months; and a *reorganization phase* that begins after the eighth month and is in process at 12 months. (Mercer, 1986, p. 300)

The three levels at which adaptation occurs are the biological, the psychological and the social. The biological level includes the woman's physical recovery and her adaptation to the growth and development of the infant. The psychological is concerned with the woman's reactions to and perceptions of being a mother, and the social is concerned with changes in her life and social relationships over the first year. During the course of the year the achievement of adaptation at the different levels varies as shown in Figure 6.4. In the physical recovery phase, the biological level predominates, while at later phases the social or psychological levels predominate. The point is made that adaptation at later phases may be inhibited if there are unresolved problems from earlier phases – for example, poor physical health in the achievement phase will inhibit the psychological and social achievements which should be occurring then.

The data demonstrate the existence of these levels and phases which have implications for practice, which Mercer (1986) describes as starting before birth with information to the woman about what to expect in labour and postnatally. Interventions are described which may assist in each of the phases. In the achievement phase, for example, Mercer (1986) notes that women need to be advised to have an examination if they have any physical or psychological problems. She found that at four months more women reported health problems than at one month postpartum. Two-thirds of the women reported health problems, 44 per cent had one problem and 22 per cent had two problems. While

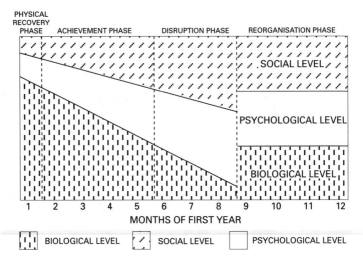

Figure 6.4   *A representation of Mercer's model of adaption to the maternal role in the first year of motherhood*

25 per cent had colds, other problems reported included genital-tract infections, chronic illnesses, gastro-intestinal problems, breast problems, joint or muscle problems, emotional tension or headaches, loss of hair, anaemia, injuries and accidents (Mercer, 1986, pp. 164–5). These findings are congruent with the findings reported by MacArthur *et al.* (1991), in Birmingham, of the high level of postnatal morbidity women experience after the six-week check. MacArthur *et al.* (1991) suggest, as does Mercer (1986), that antenatal prevention of some of these problems may be achieved, and the need to follow-up women possibly at six months post-delivery.

Mercer does not make explicit her definitions of person, health, the environment and nursing/midwifery, but the models that she has developed contain elements which indicate her thinking about these core concepts (Bee and Oetting, 1989). Health is a central concern, discussed above, in the model of antenatal stress. Similarly, the importance of the effect of factors in the social and other environment surrounding the woman are elements in the model of role attainment discussed above. In relation to the person, an assumption underlying her theory of maternal role attainment is that the woman has 'a relatively stable "core self", acquired through lifelong socialization', which determines how a mother defines and perceives events; her perceptions of her infant's and others' responses to her mothering, along with her life situation, are the real world she responds to. (Bee and Oetting, 1989, p. 297)

The role of the midwife which emerges from Mercer's writings is to assist the woman with the work needed to adjust to the maternal role and to identify and intervene where there are factors which are affecting maternal role attainment or contributing to antenatal stress.

This discussion of the work of Ramona T. Mercer has shown the process of theory development, testing and application of the theory and research results in practice. Mercer's work has been widely used, tested and adapted. Dunnington and Glazer (1991), for example, have studied the differences in role perceptions and maternal identity between mothers who were initially infertile and those who were not infertile and Pridham and Chang (1992) have undertaken a study of the problem-solving skills of women in the first three months of the infant's life. Rhoades (1989) illustrates the use that researchers have made of the data-collection tools Mercer has developed in a study which examined the degree of support provided by different people in the woman's environment on the birth of a first baby. Bee and Oetting (1989) cite McBride's assessment of Mercer's contribution to theory development which may be the best way to bring to a close this discussion of her work:

McBride wrote: 'Dr Mercer is the one who developed the most complete theoretical framework for studying one aspect of the parental experience, namely, the factors that influence the attainment of the maternal role in the first year of motherhood.' (Bee and Oetting, 1989, pp. 300–1)

ELA-JOY LEHRMAN: COMPONENTS OF MIDWIFERY PRACTICE

In Britain and elsewhere there is a considerable body of research which has examined the content and process of antenatal care (Field, 1990). Robinson *et al.* (1983, and Robinson 1985), in a study of the role of the midwife, provide comprehensive information on the clinical and advisory tasks that midwives undertake, such as abdominal examinations or providing advice on lactation and health care in pregnancy. This study was concerned with demonstrating the extent to which midwives were able to exercise all aspects of their role for care of the childbearing woman. Macintyre (1980) observed antenatal care and has demonstrated the difference between the official rhetoric about the value of antenatal care and the type of impersonal care that women experienced in a specialist obstetric unit. Concern about the lack of relationship between identification of risk factors and the effectiveness of antenatal care in relation to the physical outcomes of pregnancy led to the extensive work in Aberdeen on patterns of antenatal care (Hall *et al.*, 1985).

What Lehrman (1981) has done is take a step backwards to identify the concepts underlying the antenatal care being provided.

In Chapter 2, Hayward's (1975) model, which relates together the concepts of information, anxiety and pain, was considered. To study these concepts, Hayward had to identify measurable indicators, such as use of analgesia or the degree of pain shown on a scale, which would provide information about the amount of anxiety or pain being experienced by the individual. Robinson *et al.* (1983) were concerned in their study with role responsibilities and the questionnaires contained questions providing information about indicators of midwives' responsibilities. This type of quantitative information is vital in monitoring and developing midwifery practice but there is also a need to understand the pictures of care or concepts of care that a midwife is putting into practice, whatever the level of responsibility for care the midwife is able to exercise.

It is these underlying concepts that Lehrman (1981) and Morton *et al.* (1991) have examined in their research. If an understanding of the concepts held by midwives were combined with the information from studies such as those of Robinson *et al.* (1983), it might be possible to describe the qualitative differences in care experienced by women and the quantitative extent to which midwives are able to put the concepts of midwifery care into practice. Lehrman (1981) is asking the question: what is it that makes midwifery care important? Robinson *et al.* (1983) are saying that if midwifery care is important, the question is: to what extent are midwives able to exercise that care in practice?

Lehrman (1981) is an American nurse-midwife and her study is of the work of certified nurse-midwives. Interestingly, her data is of antenatal visits of women to nurse-midwives who are all undertaking what would be termed, in Britain, midwife-led clinics. The underlying question of her study is: 'what are the components of prenatal care provided by certified nurse-midwives?' (Lehrman, 1981, p. 27).

Lehrman developed her concepts of the components of nurse-midwifery practice through a combination of inductive and deductive theorising. Three antenatal visits were audiotaped and from these she developed initial categories or concepts of practice. This is an approach to developing theory termed grounded theory which was developed by Glaser and

Strauss (1967) (Field and Morse, 1985). In addition, Lehrman examined literature covering the preceding 25 years, which had been written by nurse-midwives: 'These articles contained a consistent reoccurrence of concepts considered to be aspects of nurse-midwifery practice. These were extracted from the literature and grouped, resulting in eight aspects of nurse-midwifery practice.' (Lehrman, 1981, p. 29).

The eight concepts describe the underlying philosophy which appears (from the literature and the grounded theory work undertaken by Lehrman) to underpin nurse-midwifery practice in antenatal care in the USA. To assess whether these concepts could be demonstrated in practice Lehrman defined and described the concepts in measurable terms (operationalised the concepts). The eight concepts are:

Continuity of care
Family-centred care
Education and counselling as part of care
Non-interventionist care
Flexibility in care
Participative care
Consumer advocacy
Time.

Taking participative care (or, in terms more familiar to British midwives, control and choice on the part of the woman) as an example, this is defined as: 'The joint assessment, evaluation, and planning of a program by the client and the health care provider.' (Lehrman, 1981, p. 29). The operational definition of this concept is:

The occurrence during the taped visit, of at least one incident of mutual collaboration on a matter between the CNM [Certified Nurse-Midwife] and client to reach a decision or conclusion; or, the occurrence of one instance where the client is involved in and /or takes responsibility for a portion of her health care during the visit. (Lehrman, 1981, pp. 29–30)

While it may be felt that this definition provides a minimum standard of participation, nevertheless the definition provides clear criteria against which observed care or data can be compared. Lehrman examined the eight concepts through the collection of data in the form of 40 audiotapes of antenatal clinic care carried out by 23 nurse-midwives which were then analysed quantitatively to measure the occurrence of these concepts in practice. The antenatal visits (none of which were booking visits) lasted an average 23.7 minutes. Table 6.1 shows Lehrman's findings in relation to the eight concepts.

The data analysis shows that these theoretical concepts or components of midwifery care were observable and occurred in the majority of the antenatal visits examined in the research. Questions may be asked about the way that some of the concepts have been operationalised. For example, the concept of time identifies the midwife as being unhurried, but 'being unhurried' is not measured by a straight measure of the length of the visit. Similarly, to measure continuity by evidence of one reference to past or future care may not adequately demonstrate the existence of 'The provision of health care which conforms in the past, present and future to the individual client's needs (Lehrman, 1981, p. 29). As Lehrman comments, longitudinal research over the whole period of pregnancy would provide a better measure of the concepts.

In the analysis, Lehrman provides information on the topics and activities covered in the visits and the lengths of time during the visits that the nurse-midwife, pregnant woman and others present at the visit were talking and asking questions. Relationships were also found between some of the components of the visits.

Table 6.1   *Analysis of the aspects of nurse-midwifery practice content categories*

Aspect	Visits where present (%)	Mean for visits where present (min.)	Mean for all visits (min.)
Time	100.0	23.7	23.7
Continuity of care	97.5	1.2	1.1
Education and counselling with care	82.5	6.0	4.9
Non-interventionist care	52.5	1.7	0.9
Participative care	47.5	1.6	0.8
Flexibility in care	42.5	1.5	0.6
Consumer advocacy	30.0	1.9	0.6
Family-centred care[*]	72.5	2.5	1.9

[*]Measured in frequency of occurrence/visit rather than duration.
(Extracted from: Table 3, Analysis of the aspects of nurse-midwifery practice content categories, Lehrman, 1981, p. 32.)

There also seemed to be a relationship between the physical examination and participative care, where the nurse-midwife would have
the woman palpate the felt parts or the significant other listen to the
fetal heartbeat. (Lehrman, 1981, p. 36)

This type of relationship has important consequences when considered with the finding that hospital midwives in consultant obstetric
units reported that 33.4 per cent of abdominal examinations were
carried out by doctors only, thus inhibiting the midwife's opportunity
for encouraging participatory care (Robinson *et al.*, 1983).

In this study, Lehrman has identified eight components or concepts
underlying nurse-midwifery care in the USA and has demonstrated the
presence of these concepts in practice. The mean duration of some of
the components in the observed visits may appear very short, but this
may be a feature of the way the components were operationalised. By
identifying these concepts and confirming the presence of the concepts
in practice, Lehrman provides a means of examining the outcomes of
antenatal care in relation to the components or underlying concepts of
that care. For example, questions which may now be asked include:
what is the relation between flexibility in care and the physical, social
and psychological outcomes of midwifery care? Is there a relationship
between participative care and outcomes? By describing these concepts
in measurable terms these relationships can be examined. Putting these
concepts into terms more familiar in Britain, questions can be asked
about the choice (flexibility), control (participative care) and continuity
(continuity of care) experienced by a woman, and the social, psychological and physical outcomes of this care. What consequences do the
eight concepts identified earlier have for the actions of midwives and
the outcomes of care experienced by the woman, her baby and family?

Morten and colleagues (Morten *et al.*, 1991) have undertaken research which examines the concepts described by Lehrman in postnatal
care. They comment,

> She categorised these as content components because, although some
> might consider these to be aspects of process, these attitudes philo-
> sophically direct what is done with the client. This distinction
> seemed unique to anything yet found in the literature and, even in
> current review, remains as such. (Morten *et al.*, 1991, p. 277).

In this study, postnatal visits were tape-recorded and analysed for evidence of the eight components. Aspects of all eight components were
identified and three additional components were identified from the
data: therapeutic techniques; empowerment; and lateral relationship.

These concepts were defined and operationalised as follows: 'therapeutic techniques were conceptually defined as a process of communication that benefits and/or encourages growth and healing' (Morten *et al.*, 1991, p. 281). Therapeutic techniques were measured by evidence (indicators) of 'active listening, probing, clarification, humour, nonjudgmental attitude, encouragement, facilitation and permission-giving' (p. 281).

Lateral relationship is defined as: 'the CNM promoting an interaction characterised by a sense of openness, mutual regard, and equal footing with the client, thus encouraging a sense of commonality between the two' (Morten *et al.*, 1991, p. 281). Lateral relationship was indicated thus: 'alignment, empathy and shared experiences and/or feelings were seen to be conducive to and representative of a lateral relationship' (p. 281).

The definition of empowerment describes empowerment as: 'the process of giving and/or receiving power, strength and ego reinforcement' (p. 281) which was demonstrated: 'when the CNM, through her attitude and approach to care, enhanced the client's inner energies and resources' (Morten *et al.*, 1991, p. 281). Evidence from the data which indicated empowerment were statements of 'affirmation, validation, reassurance and support' (p. 281).

The authors consider that the eight concepts identified by Lehrman provide a broad conceptual framework and that the three process concepts of empowerment, therapeutic techniques and lateral relationship provide greater specificity as to the process by which the broader concepts (for example, of non-interventionist care), are translated into practice. The three process components are related to and inform each other and are related to and inform the eight components identified by Lehrman. Lehrman has demonstrated some of these relationships but further research is needed. Figure 6.5 shows that each concept in this model influences the midwife and informs the care (the actions). The care experienced by the women within this model should contain evidence of the eleven components. Considering this model, it is interesting to speculate whether the care arrow may be two-way: whether a woman experiencing flexible, non-interventionist care shows empathy, empowerment and lateral relationships with midwives caring for her and whether this model is mutually reinforcing.

The work of Lehrman and Morten and colleagues provides a model of midwifery practice. This is in contrast to the work of Rubin and Mercer in which the models are focused on the women and role development. Lehrman and Morten *et al.* provide a model which clearly indicates areas of midwifery activity. In the models developed by Mercer and Rubin,

151

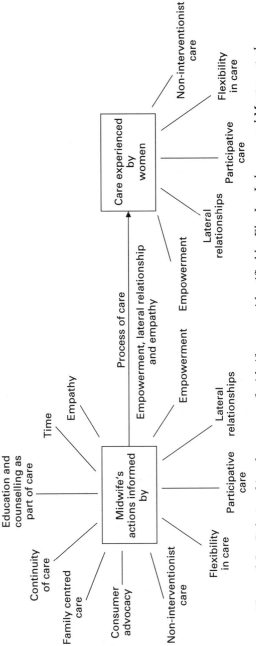

Figure 6.5   *Relationship of concepts of midwifery care identified by Ela-Joy Lehrman and Morten, et al.*

midwifery practice has to be deduced. For example, it can be deduced that to support the woman in mimicracy activities relating to nutrition, the midwife has to provide information on diet in pregnancy, and support the woman in undertaking that activity (mimicracy). Lehrman and Morten *et al.* provide a model of process or practice, while Mercer and Rubin provide a model of goals – for example, attainment of the maternal role. Although there is overlap between these characterisations of these groups of models they may be combined. It may be the case that maternal role development is achieved more easily within a system of midwifery care which provides family-centred care, flexibility in care, lateral relationships and the other components of practice described above. Testing of the relationships between these concepts will indicate the strength of the relationships that have been suggested.

To end this discussion of this work of Lehrman and Morten *et al.*, a small validation of one of the concepts will be described. During preparation of this book the author was asked by a group of midwifery lecturers to discuss with them theory in midwifery. As part of this discussion they were asked how they thought about midwifery care. One of the lecturers said that her view of practice was based on the concept of unconditional positive regard described by Carl Rogers. Unconditional positive regard contributes to the openness and equality which Morten *et al.* (1991) describe in the lateral relationship. Morten *et al.*, in the description of the lateral, therapeutic relationship, refer to the theoretical contribution provided by Rogers (1961) to their understanding of this relationship. This description by a midwifery lecturer of her approach to care suggests that the concept of lateral relationship, with its unconditional positive regard, may not be unfamiliar to midwives in Britain. The other lecturers expressed some surprise at the verbalisation by their colleague of this concept of care. Although they all work together they were unaware that their colleague approached care in the light of this model. The process of verbalisation of concepts and sharing of models of care may be less familiar in Britain than in the USA. This small incident shows that the concepts held by British midwives may not be so different from those of their American equivalents even though they are called nurse-midwives!

Lehrman (1988) has also undertaken work on the development of a middle-range theory of nurse-midwifery practice, the Nurse-Midwifery Practice Model. In the discussion of the rationale for development of this model, Lehrman (1988) identifies the lack of a theoretical base for midwifery practice and the need for midwives to move away from physical outcomes as the measures of midwifery practice. Middle-range, predictive theories, as discussed in Chapter 2, are considered to have greater relevance to practice than the grand theories or models.

The concepts which are incorporated into this theory are based on the philosophy of the American College of Nurse-Midwives, a review of the literature, Lehrman's own practice, conversations with childbearing women and nurse-midwives and preparatory research work. The Nurse-Midwifery Practice Model is a 'six-stage, five-level, multi-variate causal model encompassing the scope of nurse-midwifery practice' (Lehrman, 1988, p. 26). The scope of the model is the whole of nurse-midwifery practice. Lehrman (1988) comments that research is now required, to test the relationships between concepts that the model identifies.

In her doctoral research, Lehrman (1988) has taken the part of the model which is concerned with care in labour (one level of care) and 'Testing of the maternal psychosocial variables from the Intrapartum Care Level of the Nurse-Midwifery Practice Model was the focus of this research.' (Lehrman, 1988, p. 38). The research produced a large amount of data, some supporting and some refuting the proposed relationships in the model. As Lehrman (1988) comments: 'Of particular importance is the strong support for the concept of positive presence and the contribution of nurse-midwifery care to women's satisfaction with their labor and birth experiences as well as feelings of enhanced self-concept' (Lehrman, 1988, p. 131). This work provides food for thought for others involved in the development of midwifery theory and it is unfortunate that it has not yet been published, which would make it more accessible to midwives (Lehrman, 1993).

ERNESTINE WIEDENBACH AND THE NEED-FOR-HELP

Ernestine Wiedenbach is a nurse theorist who qualified as a nurse-midwife in her forties. She is probably most familiar from her collaborative work with the philosophers Dickoff and James in the 1960s (Dickoff *et al.*, 1992a and b). Her work with Dickoff and James took place while she was a member of the faculty of the Yale University School of Nursing, where she developed a graduate-level course in nurse-midwifery. She is identified as one of the earliest nurse theorists, and at Yale worked with other early developers of nursing theory, including Ida Orlando and Virginia Henderson (Raleigh, 1989; Nickel *et al.*, 1992). Nickel *et al.* (1992) provide a fascinating description of Wiedenbach's professional life and her conceptualisation of family-centred maternity nursing.

Wiedenbach qualified as a nurse in 1925 and worked as a nurse in various fields and as a professional writer for the Nursing Information Bureau for 20 years. She then qualified as a nurse-midwife in 1946 and worked in clinical practice until she was appointed to Yale in 1952. Nickel *et al.* (1992) comment that during the late 1940s Wiedenbach worked on a project to provide childbirth preparation based on the theories of Dr Grantley Dick-Read.

In discussions of Wiedenbach's contribution to nursing theory the emphasis is placed on her book *Clinical Nursing: A Helping Art* (1964). However, in 1958 she was the author of *Family-Centred Maternity Nursing* which she wrote because there were no textbooks which focused on the family. Incidentally, she was writing this book in the 1950s when Margaret Myles was writing and revising her influential British text. It appears that the comments of Dickoff and James on this textbook stimulated her thinking about theory (Nickel *et al.*, 1992). Wiedenbach is considered to have developed her theory inductively from experience and observation of practice (Danko *et al.*, 1989). Although she had worked for 20 years as a nurse, the development of this theory took place while she was working in the field of maternity care.

In the preface to the second edition of *Family-Centred Maternity Nursing*, Wiedenbach (1967) summarises her theory of nursing (midwifery):

> The theory of accountability which underlies the concept of nursing presented in this book, envisions the nurse as accountable not only for what she does, but also in large measure for the results she obtains from what she does. Her responses, other than reflex, according to this theory, stem from her perception of the realities which make up the situation in which she finds herself at any given point in time. Assumptions resulting from her perception and the degree of validity she attaches to them, colour the character of her responses and determine not only her immediate action but also, to a large degree, the kind of response she obtains from the recipient of her act. (Wiedenbach, 1967, p. v)

This broad conceptual model encompasses five elements which Wiedenbach terms the Realities of Nursing:

> the agent: (the nurse, midwife or other person)
> the recipient: (the woman, family, community)
> the goal: the goal of the intervention
> the means: the method to reach the goal
> the framework: the social, organisational and professional environment (Wiedenbach, 1967, pp. 5–6)

The relationships between the Realities of Nursing are illustrated in Figure 6.6. These elements are elaborated in discussions of Wiedenbach's other work.

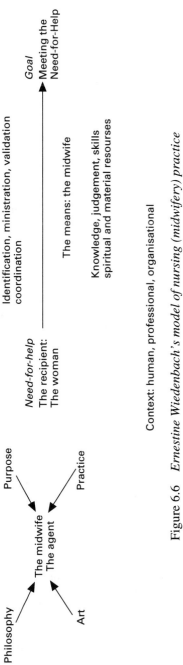

Figure 6.6 *Ernestine Wiedenbach's model of nursing (midwifery) practice*

1.   The Agent – the midwife

Raleigh (1989) cites Wiedenbach's (1964) identification of 'four elements in clinical nursing: (i) philosophy, (ii) purpose, (iii) practice and
(iv) art' (p. 91). She states that nursing is based on an explicit philosophy and describes three points that are basic to a philosophy of nursing.

a.   Reverence for the gift of life.
b.   Respect for the dignity, worth, autonomy and individuality of
     each human being.
c.   Resolution to act dynamically in relation to one's beliefs.
     (Raleigh, 1989, p. 91)

Raleigh (1989) comments that it cannot be assumed that all practitioners hold the same philosophy, but this model is helpful in identifying
the need to consider the beliefs of the individual midwife and the
beliefs of colleagues. In relation to midwifery Wiedenbach's (1967)
own philosophy of midwifery care and action is demonstrated in her
description of the 'ultimate goal of maternity nursing'(p. 22), which

> extends beyond the immediate needs of the mother and baby, to the
> broader needs of the mother and father to develop inner strengths –
> Power in Reserve – on which to draw with confidence and under-
> standing as they prepare for and assume their roles of parents.
> (Wiedenbach, 1967, p. 22).

2.   The Goal/Purpose

The goal or purpose of the nurse, according to Wiedenbach, is to meet a
person's need-for-help. Danko *et al.* (1989) cite Wiedenbach's (1964)
definition of a need-for-help: 'A need-for-help is "any measure or
action required and desired by the individual and which has potential
for restoring or extending his ability to cope with the demands implicit
in his situation"' (Danko *et al.*, 1989, p. 241).

Needs have to be recognised by the nurse or midwife and, according
to this model, must be acknowledged by the individual. Danko *et al.*
(1989) comment that this restricts the use of the model as, for example,
an infant or comatose person cannot recognise or express a need-for-
help. However, Wiedenbach (1967) illustrates the utility of this idea in
midwifery practice in a description of the identification of postnatal
needs:

> Whenever a need-for-help exists, its presence may usually be sus-
> pected by behaviour – physical, emotional or physiological – which

is different from the normal or usual pattern. The nurse [midwife] who is perceptive will be aware of it. Perceptiveness thus is an important attribute of postpartum nursing. The fact that a need is perceived, however, does not mean that it is met. First it must be identified. To do this requires skilled use of eyes, ears, hands and mind – eyes through which to observe or look intently; ears with which to listen expectantly; hands with which to feel, touch or palpate sensitively; and a mind with which to understand and interpret the observation. Once the need is recognised and has been validated by the one whose need it is, appropriate action may be taken to meet it. (Wiedenbach, 1967, pp. 353–4)

3. The Recipient

The recipient of care may be the childbearing woman, the family or the community, who, for some reason or another are unable to meet their present needs. Nickel *et al.* (1992) comment that Wiedenbach's philosophy emphasises her respect for the individual. Raleigh (1989) summarises Wiedenbach's view of the recipient:

The individual is seen as competent and able to determine if a need-for-help is being experienced. Nurses need to intervene only when there is an obstacle preventing the individual from satisfactorily coping with the demands placed upon him or her by the situation. (Raleigh, 1989, p. 92)

4. The Means

The means of achieving the goal of midwifery care are expressed in practice which comprises four phases:

(i)   *Identification* of the patient's experienced need-for-help.
(ii) *Ministration* of the help that is needed.
(iii) *Validation* that the help provided was indeed the help needed.
(iv) *Co-ordination* of the resources for help provided. (Raleigh, 1989, p. 91–2)

The model identifies the need for the midwife to have knowledge, judgement and skills to enable the above steps of care to be achieved:

Knowledge encompasses everything that has been comprehended. *Judgement* involves the ability of the nurse to make sound decisions. *Skills* represent the nurse's ability to achieve the appropriate outcomes. (Raleigh, 1989, p. 91)

In meeting the individual's need-for-help the nurse or midwife demonstrates the art of nursing or midwifery. This artistry is illustrated in the above description of the identification of needs and is a result of the combination of observation and intuition with knowledge:

> In an attempt to further clarify the concept [art], Wiedenbach states that it is comprised of deliberative action that seems to be based on intuition. This is a professional intuition influenced by knowledge and judgment. She states that, prior to deliberative action, the nurse analyzes information based on perceptions and feelings and the exercise of judgment, while keeping in mind the overall purpose with respect to the patient. (Raleigh, 1989, p. 96)

Wiedenbach developed her model of the Helping Art of Nursing inductively from her nursing and nurse-midwifery practice. The model helps to identify components of midwifery/nursing practice which contribute to the goals of care. This type of model, which focuses on practice rather than outcome, can be likened to the model of midwifery practice developed by Lehrman (1981). Wiedenbach's central concern is with the influence of the knowledge, attitudes and theories held by midwives (and nurses) on practice. Danko *et al.* (1989) suggest that Wiedenbach's concepts are currently being applied to nursing practice to a greater extent than they were in the 1950s and 1960s. They refer to an article that Wiedenbach wrote in 1949, in which she described the type of natural childbirth that women wanted, and comment: 'But not until the 1970s were some or most of these needs for help met. In the 1980s the health care industry provided the supposedly unique concept of Family Centred Care, which Wiedenbach addressed some 20 years ago.' (Danko *et al.*, 1989, p. 249).

Wiedenbach made a significant contribution to the development of midwifery theory and in drawing out and helping to explain the different factors which contribute to skilled practice. This skilled, knowledgeable, creative practice in which the midwife coordinates care to meet the needs of the woman and her family is described and illustrated with numerous case studies in *Family-Centred Maternity Nursing*. Her model helps in the discussion of underlying theory which she identified as vital: 'she would stress that only through thoughtful and systematic exploration of our beliefs and intents can the way be found to improve nursing practice'(Nickel *et al.*, 1992, p. 166). She believed that theory is 'inextricably interlocked with practice, it underlies it and is responsible for its character and quality' (Wiedenbach, cited by Nickel *et al.*, 1992, p. 166).

JEAN BALL – THE DECK-CHAIR THEORY OF MATERNAL EMOTIONAL WELL-BEING

Jean Ball, a British midwife, has undertaken extensive research into the postnatal needs of women and the consequences for women of different forms of organisation of maternity services (Ball, 1981; 1987; 1989). In *Reactions to Motherhood* (1987) she describes the following aim of postnatal care:

> The purpose of all maternity care is to enable a woman to be successful in becoming a mother, and this success applies not only to the physiological processes involved but also to the psychological and emotional processes which motivate the desire for parenthood and its fulfilment. (Ball, 1987, p. 127)

This aim can be seen as Ball's personal aim or philosophy of postnatal care. If the continuum shown in Figure 5.1 is considered, it is possible to locate Ball's position. In practice, in many organisations, the type of care provided may be closer to an obstetric/medical model of pregnancy within which interest in postnatal care is minimal (as delivery has been achieved), and postnatal care continues to be the Cinderella of care of the childbearing woman.

The description above identifies pregnancy and the postnatal period as a time of adoption of a new role. The literature review for Ball's (1987) study of postnatal care identifies role theory, change theory, theories of stress, coping and support as the theoretical basis for the study. The concepts investigated are drawn from theories of coping and support systems and the variables investigated relate to the woman's personality, life-events and personal and family circumstances, factors relating to the birth and progress following the birth and the woman's views of care, support and emotional well-being.

The hypotheses for the study were that:

> The emotional response of women to the changes which follow the birth of a child will be affected by their personality and by the quality of support they receive from family and social support systems. The way in which care is provided by midwives during the postnatal period will influence the emotional response of women to the changes which follow the birth of a child. (Ball, 1987, p. 37)

The variables were investigated through collection of information from 279 women. The data were collected using structured interviews administered antenatally, in the early postnatal period and by a postal questionnaire at six weeks. The information from the women was supplemented with interview data from the midwives who were responsible for transferring the women home, and postal questionnaire data from the community midwives involved with the women. The data were analysed quantitatively to identify those factors which affected the women's emotional well-being and their satisfaction with motherhood. The factors which were found to contribute to emotional well-being are shown in Figure 6.7. Ball (1987) comments:

> Good scores on all these factors would result in a high degree of emotional wellbeing, while poor scores on all of them would result in considerable distress. But as these factors also interact with each other, if poor scores on certain factors are counterbalanced by good scores on others, it might be possible for the potential emotional outcome to be improved. (Ball, 1987, p. 118).

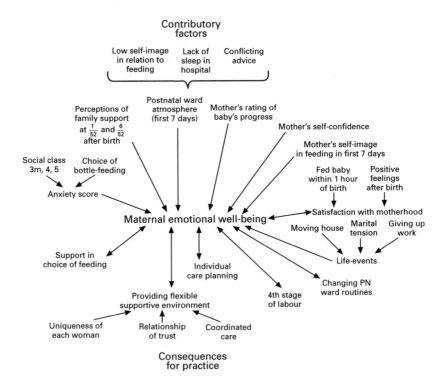

Figure 6.7   *Factors identified by Jean Ball as affecting maternal emotional well-being*

The analysis supported both hypotheses of the study which indicated that a woman's well-being following delivery is dependent on her own personality, her personal support system and the support provided by the maternity services. Ball (1987) illustrates the interrelationship of these three elements as a deck-chair, as shown in Figure 6.8. The base of the chair is formed by the maternity services resting on the views of society regarding families, the side-strut of the woman's personality, life experiences, and so on, and the central strut her family and support system. The woman's maternal well-being (the seat of the chair) is dependent on the effective coming together of all these elements:

> If a deckchair is not erected properly, it will collapse under the weight of its occupant; if it does not stand on a firm base it will fall

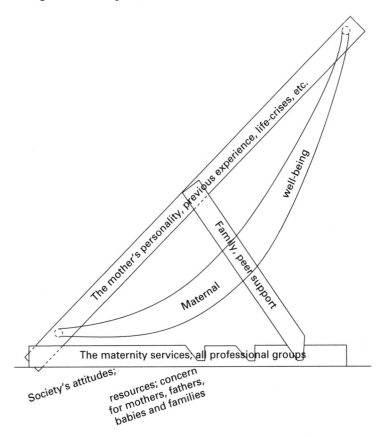

Figure 6.8   *Support systems for maternal well-being*

(Ball, 1987, Fig. 7.1, p. 121 reproduced with permission of Cambridge University Press)

over with similar results; and if the parts do not fit together well the occupant may be held up, but will become uncomfortable and strained. (Ball, 1987, p. 120)

The deckchair can be seen to have similarities to the action framework where the views of society, the individual's definition of the situation and the organisation of services all contribute to the action – the woman's maternal well-being (see Chapter 3). Interesting parallels can also be drawn between Ball's work and that of Mercer (1986). In addition, if the picture or theory of maternal well-being that Ball has identified, from empirical data in combination with a theoretical framework, is compared with the key concepts of midwifery described in Chapter 2, it can be seen that this theory addresses each of these of concepts.

Women – the focus of Ball's work is concern for individual women and for their successful emotional, social and psychological development during the childbirth process;

Health – health is central to this model, being seen in the definition of the aim of postnatal care: 'to enable a woman to be successful in becoming a mother' (Ball, 1987, p. 127).

Environment – the social and organisational environments in the form of support systems and postnatal care services (as well as the wider society) are important elements of this model, support having been shown to be crucial for the well-being of the woman.

Midwifery – in part the research on postnatal care was motivated by a concern about the lack of information about the effects of midwifery care on emotional well-being. The model provides guidance on many areas of intervention by midwives which are discussed by Ball, including patterns of care, support in decisions on feeding methods, help with feeding and individual care planning (see Figure 6.7).

Self – the theory clearly starts from the standpoint that the role of the midwife is to support and assist the woman to become confident in the role of mother. Ball (1987) contends that services and patterns of care must change in response to the needs of women, however painful that may be for the health professionals concerned. The stance underpinning this approach to care is thus one of listening, learning and changing.

This theory relates together concepts of, for example, anxiety, life-events and emotional well-being and can be described as a factor-relating theory (Dickoff *et al.*, 1992, see Chapter 2) and the relationships between the factors, or concepts, now need to be tested further by research. In addition, there is now a need for midwives to undertake further research to determine what aspects of midwifery practice may modify, for example, women's perceptions of the postnatal ward atmosphere or the woman's self-image of feeding in the first seven days. It is time to test the deckchair and Ball's Deck-Chair Theory of Maternal Emotional Wellbeing.

Summary

Within this chapter the theory building and testing which has been undertaken by four nurse-midwives and one midwife have been presented. The focus of Rubin's and Mercer's research has been the process by which women attain the maternal role. Clarification of this process provides indicators of ways in which midwives and others can assist women in this process. These models clearly identify childbearing as a social rather than medical process. The models developed by Lehrman and Wiedenbach put more emphasis on understanding the process of nurse-midwifery intervention. Lehrman, in addition, appears to be the first nurse-midwife to have developed a grand or general theory of nurse-midwifery practice.

Ball's work has been aimed at providing information about factors which contribute to emotional well-being in the postnatal period. The support system model which has been generated as a result of her research identifies many concepts. This model now requires further development and refinement through further research. The four American theorists in this chapter all demonstrate the effectiveness of research programmes conducted over many years. Rubin's work, for example, is based on the research observations of many research students over 25 years. It is possible that the lack of such programmes of research in Britain may be one of the factors which has contributed to the dearth of theory development in British midwifery.

Activities

Use these activities to reflect on the relevance of this chapter for your own practice.

1 Describe the main concepts in the model of maternal role attainment proposed by Rubin. What relevance do these concepts have for your practice?
2 Describe the main concepts in the model of maternal role attainment proposed by Mercer. What relevance do these concepts have for your practice?
3 What are the essential differences and similarities in the models described by Rubin and Mercer?

4 What consequences do the eight concepts identified by Lehrman (1981) have for the actions of midwives and the outcomes of care experienced by the woman, her baby and family?

5 Describe the main concepts in the model of care proposed by Wiedenbach. What relevance do these concepts have for your practice?

6 Consider the model of postnatal support proposed by Ball. In what ways does care in the setting in which you work facilitate or inhibit maternal well-being through attention to the elements identified by Ball?

7 In what ways are the concepts identified by these authors the same as or different from the concepts that form the basis for your practice?

8 How could you implement one of these models (if appropriate) into the care of the childbearing woman?

CHAPTER SEVEN

Approaches to theory building in midwifery

Working as 'skilled companion' to the woman, the midwife should combine clinical skills and scientific knowledge with a sensitivity to this significant event: the start of a new life. In accompanying the woman and her partner on the journey to parenthood, midwives should help women to exercise choice and control over their bodies and the birth of their babies. By renewing approaches to practice while drawing on tradition, we may find promise in the future of the profession for women, families and midwives. (Page, 1993, p. 24)

INTRODUCTION

Considerable work has been undertaken on the development of theory for midwifery and there is a growing body of literature on which to draw when theory in midwifery is being developed. However, while there is a considerable body of work by American nurse-midwives, there is less evidence of theory building in midwifery than in nursing. The development of models for midwifery practice has not occurred to any great extent although, as discussed earlier, midwifery care is based on a wide range of theories, and significant work has been done by a number of people to identify the midwifery concepts underpinning practice. This lack of development contrasts with the picture in nursing. Fitzpatrick and Whall (1989) discuss the work of 25 nurse theorists of whom only one (Wiedenbach) has undertaken significant work in the field of midwifery. In addition to Wiedenbach, Marriner-Tomey (1989) includes a discussion of the work of Mercer, an American nurse-midwife, in a description of the work of 28 nurse theorists.

This lack of specific theory development in British midwifery is confirmed by the dearth of literature on the subject. The MIDIRS (Midwives Information and Resource Service) reference list on

'Midwifery Models and Midwifery Process' (1992) contains 48 references. However, while this list contains articles on the use of models in midwifery (for example, Morton *et al.*, 1991; Smith, 1991) it also contains references to systems (models) of organising care (for example, Waterhouse, 1989; Currell 1990), education (for example, Leong, 1989) and use of the midwifery/nursing process (for example, Kesby and Grant, 1985; Bryar, 1987). The select reading list from the Royal College of Midwives entitled 'Nursing and Midwifery Models' contained 41 items, 13 of which relate directly to midwifery practice but several of these are concerned with models in general rather than models for midwifery care. The database at the Royal College of Nursing yielded only eight items under the heading of midwifery models.

Interest in the use of models in midwifery began in the early 1980s in Britain, stimulated by a concern to provide more individualised care and to meet the wider needs of women as well as a concern to demonstrate and express the full role of the midwife. Initially attempts to achieve individualised care were focused on the use of the nursing/midwifery process (Whitfield, 1983; Adams *et al.*, 1981) and birth plans (Carty and Tier, 1989). During the late 1980s and early 1990s attention has been focused on achieving individualised care through a continuous relationship with a named midwife and various forms of team midwifery (Department of Health, 1993a; Flint, 1993). Interest in understanding how midwives think and how their pictures of practice affect midwifery care has developed during the past ten years on a number of fronts:

(i)   identification of philosophies of care (see Chapter 5);
(ii)   adaptation of nursing models to midwifery;
(iii)   development of local models;
(iv)   quality assurance developments.

Before developments in (ii)–(iv) are considered, the effect of the nursing/midwifery process on the development of models in midwifery in Britain will be discussed.

NURSING/MIDWIFERY PROCESS

Midwives have expressed concern about the use of models in midwifery. Part of this concern, Henderson (1990) argues, stems from the introduction of the nursing/midwifery process prior to discussion and development of models. The nursing/midwifery process is a logical approach to the assessment and identification of needs and problems, planning to meet those needs and evaluating the effectiveness of the actions taken prior to reassessment to identify new needs or problems, and is defined as follows: 'Planned individualised midwifery care is a logical, systematic approach to the total care of a mother, baby and family unit. It includes the following steps: a) assessing, b) planning, c) implementing and d) evaluating' (Bradshaw and Whitfield, 1986, p. 1).

Pearson and Vaughan (1986) provide a graphic representation of the interrelationship of models and the nursing process. They describe the model as a series of 'goals' that are transported to a patient via a vehicle – the nursing process. In addition they make the point that the nursing process or problem-solving approach to care is not unique to nursing, but is a tool used in many professions and in day-to-day life, for example, when planning a holiday. What makes nursing unique are the values and models which are transmitted by the nursing process vehicle or tool to the patient and similarly what makes midwifery unique are the values and models that are transmitted to the childbearing woman.

If early reports of the introduction of the nursing/midwifery process are examined, it is evident that discussion of the underlying beliefs and values of the midwives were held even if these discussions did not lead to the identification of specific models. Whitfield (1983) describes concerns held by women, which underpinned the midwifery process project at the Mothers' Hospital, about lack of continuity of care, conflicting advice, lack of information and lack of attention to social and emotional needs, and comments that the midwifery process

> acknowledges the fact that to every mother the experience of pregnancy and childbirth is unique. No one woman approaches it in exactly the same way, and the joys and difficulties that pregnancy, labour and a new baby bring will be different for each. (Whitfield, 1983, p. 186).

These statements clearly identify concepts relating to the woman, her health, midwifery practice and the goals of care, although not explicitly stated as a model. In 1979–82 the author was involved in a project which was similarly based on the issues identified by Whitfield (1983) above (Adams *et al.*, 1981; Bryar and Strong, 1983; Bryar, 1985; Bryar, 1991a). The aim of the project was to individualise the midwifery care experienced by women and, as part of this, the nursing/midwifery process tool was introduced. Discussions were held with midwives in the hospital and community about the assessment framework they needed to provide midwifery care. They had already devised a midwifery history which, in addition to the medical/obstetric history, contained information on

(i)   the social circumstances of the woman and the support available
        to her;
(ii)   the woman and her family's adjustment to the pregnancy and
        plans during the pregnancy;
(iii)   a profile of her health before she became pregnant.

Again, these areas identify the underlying concepts of care held by
the midwives. During development of the midwifery assessment,
Henderson's Activities of Daily Living (Quillin and Runk, 1989) were
included but were not used by the midwives. At the time we concluded
that this was because the midwives were being faced with a large
number of changes (to achieve individualised care) and were not able to
take on this additional change as well. The final midwifery assessment,
which accompanied the woman, from booking to discharge by the community midwives, included assessment items in the following areas:

    obstetric/medical history;
    social/family history;
    health practices during pregnancy;
    health/social work staff providing care during pregnancy.

This list indicates that the midwives involved in this study were
aware of the influence of the range of factors affecting the childbearing
woman as identified, for example, by Ball (1987), but had not got to the
stage of expressing these factors as a model of midwifery. Indeed, the
notion of a model of midwifery was not one which was discussed
widely at the time. 'No midwifery frameworks on which to base an assessment were identified in the literature by the project team, a finding
also reported by Keane (1982), although later in the project the assessment frameworks developed by Rubin (1967a and 1967b) and Josten
(1981) were considered' (Bryar, 1985, p. 143).

So, while agreeing with Henderson (1990) that the nursing/
midwifery process was introduced largely without attention to the
model of midwifery care, there is evidence that concern for the model
of practice was an implicit concern of those involved in the early use of
the nursing/midwifery process.

A second criticism of the nursing/midwifery process which
Henderson (1990) argues influenced midwives' views of models is the
orientation of the process towards problem-solving. Henderson (1990)
refers to the evidence of the Royal College of Midwives to the Nursing
Process Evaluation Group: 'The College was of the view that there
were drawbacks in the adaptation of the nursing process to midwifery
in that the problem solving approach of the nursing process was more
suited to a sickness model of care' (Hayward, 1986, p. 31).

Midwives are essentially concerned with supporting women throughout normal childbearing. This support requires the identification of needs and problems, be they physical, social, educational, psychological, economic or other, which the midwife can either meet herself or refer to someone else for advice. There is considerable evidence (see, for example, Hillan, 1992) that women consider that they have needs which are not currently being met:

> There is ample evidence in the press and from research, for example, Laryea (1980), that actual problems experienced by women are not identified at present, let alone possible problems or problems in the wider community. (Bryar, 1987, p. 112).

While there are many reasons why needs are problems and not identified, including organisational constraints and lack of interviewing skills (Methven, 1990), it may be suggested that lack of explicit exploration of values, concepts and models of care contributes to lack of identification. For example, if a midwife believes (holds the concept) that a woman should be a full partner in her care, the midwife will want to know what she knows about different systems of care and want to ascertain if she has a need for information. If, on the other hand the midwife's view (concept) of care is that the professionals should make the decisions, the midwife will not try to identify what the woman knows but will present information about the main system of care and will not identify any needs or concerns the woman might have. Once midwives have made their models of care explicit this assists in the process of understanding why certain needs may or may not be explored by those midwives. Assessment and care planning can then be seen as simply ways of translating the models of care into practice.

In their evidence, the Royal College of Midwives raise another argument against the nursing/midwifery process: that it conflicts with teamwork:

> as the care of the mother and baby did not belong to any one group of carers, the application of a process based on the contribution of one group was not appropriate. Any process of care in midwifery would need to be based on a health model and take into consideration all those professionals likely to contribute to that care. (Hayward, 1986, p. 31)

In the 1990s, there is a new emphasis on the lead professional in care of the childbearing woman but this care is still based within the context of a multidisciplinary team (Department of Health, 1993a and 1993b). Rather than conflicting with teamwork the nursing/midwifery process may be seen to contribute to teamwork by making explicit actions taken to meet identified needs by members of different professional groups.

Kesby and Grant (1985) identify this feature as a key reason for adopting the nursing/midwifery process:

> Despite this, many of us follow a system that fails to create the opportunity for choices to be made, that is inadequate in its means of passing on information from one department to another and that, in the absence of a regular evaluation of care, often perpetuates ineffective treatments and leaves problems unsolved.
>
> The underlying problem is undoubtedly communication between staff and patients, and staff with staff. To put this right two things have to change – the way we work and the records we keep. (Kesby and Grant, 1985, p. 28).

These authors argue that a logically organised set of midwifery records that are carried by the woman and used by midwives throughout the childbirth process assist the process of communication with the woman and those involved in her care.

The Royal College of Midwives (above) is arguing for the focus of care to be the woman rather than the midwife or other professional group. Currell (1990) describes the need to provide unity of care from the perspective of the woman through a clear focus as to the woman's needs or problems, and coordination of care from different members of the health team who help to meet those needs.

Another criticism that can be made of the use of the nursing/ midwifery process is the way that it has been adopted as a new ritual action in midwifery care. Midwifery is not unique in its adoption of ritual practices which can be seen as a means of imposing some order on an essentially uncertain world (Berger and Luckmann, 1967). Ritual practices in midwifery included routine shaving and enemas, the frequency of antenatal examinations and positions in labour (Romney and White, 1984; Hall *et al.*, 1985). Rather than contributing to individualised care, the midwifery process and care plans have in some instances become routinised and ritualistic as the following excerpt from the reflective diary of a lecturer in midwifery shows:

Thursday 18th April – 12 mid-day

Moira and I discussed her progress with breast feeding and drew up a plan of care for the day that would take into account her previous experience of breast feeding. She had breast fed her two previous children and therefore had vast experience which we both felt would be a valuable resource for learning.

Moira was quite pleased to see that someone was recognising her experiences and this made her feel 'useful'. I jokingly said she probably had more experience than I and could probably teach me 'a thing or two'.

Feeling pleased with my work with Moira I was about to see my next client when I was informed that there was a standard care plan for common needs identified in postnatal care. I examined the standardised plan of care and found that it was not appropriate for Moira since it did not take into consideration her previous experiences and moreover it would be a waste of resources since Moira was not experiencing any of the problems identified in this standardised care plan.

I explained to the midwife in charge my rationale for devising an individual plan of actions adding that it was crucial to the promotion of individualised client care. But whilst she accepted my explanation she informed me that it was ward policy that all care plans had to follow the standard format. It appeared that this was in case any question was raised later about the quality of client care, there would be this documentation for evidence.

In the end Moira had a standardised care plan written up for her care for the day. My reaction was one of anger and frustration at the lack of any attempt to promote individualised client-centred care. (McCrea, unpublished)

As with some of the other problems associated with use of the nursing/midwifery process discussed above, this ritualistic use is not inherent in this tool for care but has been an outcome of the way the tool has been used and thought about.

To counter some of the negative attitudes to the nursing/midwifery process, while maintaining its utility in assisting the midwife to think about care and share her plans for care with the woman and other colleagues, Tiran and Nunnerley (1986) focused on planned individualised care (PIC) (Hughes, 1988) in their introduction of COMB (Care of Mothers and Babies). COMB entailed many changes and innovations in the form of teams, flexibility and continuity of care and new record systems. The underlying philosophy of this approach is clearly stated:

The main aims of COMB are: to involve the parents fully in the care that they receive, to provide individualised care to all mothers and babies within the constraints of ward organisation; to encourage staff to plan that care with flexibility; to improve, but not increase, midwifery record keeping. (Tiran and Nunnerley, 1986, p. 208)

Planning of care is clearly seen as a small contribution to the whole, enabling midwives to think through the care they are providing.

As Hughes (1988) comments with reference to Tiran and Nunnerley (1986),

> This idea of a thinking, collaborative approach in which assessment, planning and evaluation shape the nature of intervention (or non-intervention) rather than age-old ritual or dogmatic policy, has already been taken up by midwives (Hughes, 1988, p. 2).

Mayes (1987) provides an illuminating description of the model of care devised by the midwives at Whipps Cross Hospital, London, which incorporates the nursing/midwifery process as the tool for putting the model into practice. In an interesting answer to the perennial issue that midwives do not deal with problems, the model described distinguishes between a complication or problem and health promotion needs. In the case of problems and complications: 'a) specific goals are formulated to solve each problem; b) specific midwifery care is "prescribed" for each problem; c) priorities are decided' (Mayes, 1987, p. viii).

In relation to health promotion issues, 'A plan is formulated to enable the mother to readjust and maintain health' (Mayes, 1987, p. viii). This differentiation of the two types of need being addressed by midwifery care highlights the central place of health promotion in midwifery practice.

Planned individualised care or the midwifery/nursing process is therefore a tool which can contribute to the way midwives think about care. It may be used in the most high-tech situations. For example, where a woman at high risk is being cared for with the use of monitors, any change in the fetal heart rate is noted by the midwife and forms part of the assessment information that is combined together to ascertain whether there is a need for intervention (a problem). The type of intervention needed to meet the goal of care will then be instituted and the outcome of that care evaluated and the fetal and maternal conditions reassessed. In this situation the local identification of the need and steps required to correct the problem will assist communication with team members who may need to be called upon. This approach may also be applied in the most empathetic of situations. For example, a community midwife helping a woman breast-feed may suddenly find the woman is weeping. Through listening to and holding the woman she may discover the root of the woman's despair (her need). Drawing on her experience, knowledge and skills, she will be able to respond to those needs either immediately or through contacting others who may be able to provide additional support. Again, either immediate evaluation (checking out with the woman) or later evaluation on subsequent visits will help to show whether the woman has been able to resolve her distress. So it can be seen that this process simply helps identify the steps the midwife goes through in caring for someone. How this process is used will depend upon how midwives think about care – what models they hold. As Fender (1981), Mayes (1987) and the Royal College of Midwives (Hayward, 1986) comment that this model needs to be based on health, as discussed earlier, health would appear to be a central concept in any model of midwifery practice (see Chapter 2). This process of thinking helps the midwife to assist the woman, her baby and family maintain or improve their health.

ADAPTATION OF NURSING MODELS TO MIDWIFERY

Due to the perceived lack of midwifery models of care alongside the explication of midwifery philosophies, there has been work on the adaptation to midwifery of models developed for nursing care.

In late 1987 and early 1988, Hughes and Goldstone (1989) undertook a survey of maternity units in the four countries of Great Britain. They obtained 186 responses; of these 174 responded to a question asking whether they were using or planning to use a model of care. Sixty-four units (37 per cent) responded that they were using a model, while 16 (9 per cent) were planning to use a model. They also found that 138 (77.5 per cent) of units had implemented or were implementing the midwifery process or planned individualised care, indicating that many were using this tool without having a clear shared framework or model within which to base their care. Some units were using one or more models but Table 7.1 indicates that Orem's Self-Care Theory of Nursing was the most commonly used model.

Interestingly, Hughes and Goldstone (1989) also found that, of the 64 units using a model of care only, 37 were also using the midwifery process or planned individualised care. As the four theories identified above rest on translation into practice via the process of nursing, this is a little difficult to understand but may be due to the confusion surrounding the use of these terms, as (Murphy-Black, 1992a) comments:

> As there is considerable confusion in the midwifery literature about the differences and similarities between the nursing process, the midwifery process, a nursing model or a midwifery model, the Supervisors of Midwives were asked to describe the process or model used within their units. (Murphy-Black, 1992a, p. 25)

Table 7.1 *Models used for maternity care*

	Number of units	% of 186 respondents
Orem	36	19
Roper/Logan/Tierney	15	8
Henderson	8	4
Roy	4	2
Own model	16	9
Other model*	13	7

*Examples include Saxton and Hylands, 'Crisis Intervention'; Stenhouse, 'The ENB Model' (Table 7 from Hughes and Goldstone, 1989, p. 166). (Reproduced with permission of Churchill Livingstone)

Murphy-Black (1992a; 1992b) undertook a two-stage survey of systems of care in maternity units in Scotland in 1990–91. Responses from 81 units in Scotland indicated that 53 (65.4 per cent) were using the nursing/midwifery process or a model. In phase 2 of the survey, more detailed information was obtained from 16 units. Of these, seven specified the model on which care was based, three were using Orem, three Roper, Logan and Tierney and one Roy's model (Murphy-Black, 1992a, p. 25). Thus it appears that almost 44 per cent of the 16 units were basing their care on a nursing model. No midwifery models were identified although respondents reported adapting the nursing models to midwifery. This 44 per cent finding is a slight increase on the 37 per cent of units that Hughes and Goldstone (1989) reported as using a model.

Henderson (1990) supports the view that Orem's self-care model and the model developed by Roper, Logan and Tierney (1980), which is based on 12 activities of daily living, have been the most widely used in midwifery. She comments:

> Orem's model, with its focus on 'self-care' and health, including the care of dependants, is pertinent to midwifery. Individual responsibility is valued, with health education an important aspect of care. Its underlying features are consistent with the role of the midwife, intervening where necessary (particularly during labour) but with a high supportive/educative profile during pregnancy and the postnatal period. (Henderson, 1990, p. 59)

The utility of this model in helping to identify areas of concern and areas for intervention by the midwife are clearly shown in Methven's (1986a) illustration of this model in practice (see below).

In the following, a number of nursing models which have been adapted for use in midwifery care will be discussed. In all the descriptions of the development and utilisation of these models, the authors provide information about the ways that the care process is recorded. Recording of such information is a vital part of the process of care and helps to contribute to continuity of care. In the following discussion, the systems of records are not described in detail and the reader is referred to the original for information on the record systems.

ROPER, LOGAN AND TIERNEY: ACTIVITIES OF LIVING MODEL

The Roper, Logan and Tierney Activities of Living Model of Nursing is probably the only general model of nursing which has been developed in Britain. It has been widely used in Britain partly because, as an indigenous model, it uses terms and language which are more familiar to British nurses than some of the language used by American theorists. The model is based on a model of living and was influenced by Virginia Henderson's (1969) definition of nursing (which is discussed below) and the 14 activities of daily living identified by Henderson (Roper *et al.*, 1985).

The authors argue that a model of nursing should be based on a model of living, as individuals only require nursing care intermittently in their lives. They consider that nursing should provide as little disruption to the person's life as possible and that this may be facilitated if nurses base their practice on a model which considers the individual within the context of their everyday life (Roper *et al.*, 1985, p. 63). Midwifery care is similarly intermittent and is concerned with the woman and the context within which she lives. Midwifery practice is concerned with helping the woman and her family meet their needs during the pregnancy and following the birth and integrating their new roles into their ongoing lives. A model which is based on an awareness of the woman's whole life would appear to have the possibility to assist midwifery practice.

The model comprises five elements:

the lifespan;
the activities of living;
the dependence/independence of the individual in relation to each of the activities of living;
factors influencing the activities of living: individualised nursing.

The lifespan underpins the model as it rests on the idea of the course of the person's life. The ability of individuals at different stages of their lives to meet their needs (activities of living) will be affected by their position in the lifespan.

The model identifies 12 areas that people need to address as part of the process of living. Although they are identified as separate activities, Roper *et al.* (1985) make the point that the activities are all interrelated. This interrelationship is seen, for example, in pregnancy, where the activities of eating and drinking, mobilising and eliminating are all affected by the activity of expressing sexuality. The areas are called activities of living but incorporated within each are a large number of separate activities (Roper *et al.*, 1981). The 12 activities of living are:

Maintaining a safe environment
Communicating
Breathing
Eating and drinking
Eliminating
Personal cleansing and dressing
Controlled body temperature
Mobilising
Working and playing
Expressing sexuality
Sleeping
Dying

The third element in the model is the degree of dependence or independence that the individual has in meeting each of the activities of living. Total independence and total dependence are represented as being at either end of a continuum (Roper *et al.*, 1985). The life-span and the dependence/independence continuum are interrelated, as Roper *et al.* (1985) illustrate with reference to the development of the person from infanthood through childhood to adolescence and adulthood.

Independence is clearly related to the life-span but may also be affected by other factors affecting the life of the individual. Additional factors influencing the individual comprise the fourth element in the model. Five factors are identified: physical, psychological, socio-cultural, environmental and politico-economic factors. Each of these is considered in relation to each of the activities of living which, combined, describe the life of the individual. This model can be related to the action model discussed in Chapter 3 where the factors in society comprise the five factors identified by Roper *et al.* (1985). These factors influence the individual's (the actor's) activities of living and affect the life (the action) experienced by the individual.

In the model of living on which the model of nursing is based, the person's individuality in living is the fifth element in the model and, in the model of nursing, the fifth element is the individuality of nursing care aimed at supporting the individuality of living of the person.

This model considers the individual's ability to meet their own needs within the 12 activities of living. The person's ability to meet their needs is dependent upon their age (position in the life-span) and position on the independence/dependence continuum. The model takes account of the needs of the baby who is unable to meet her or his own needs due to youth and the needs of the older adult who has failing sight and reduced independence. Dependence/independence may be affected by age, illness or the adoption of new roles, such as motherhood, as Pearson and Vaughan (1986) comment:

> Mature adults of 30 years may be at the independent end in virtually all activities of living, but may become dependent if illness or trauma occurs or if they are placed in an environment with which they are unfamiliar, for example, the middle of the Amazon jungle. (Pearson and Vaughan, 1986, p. 55)

The model provides a framework for the assessment of the woman throughout the childbearing process within which she may demonstrate ꜀ꜰpendence in some activities at some times, independence in other activities and changes in her independence in others as she adapts to her new role during the course of pregnancy, childbirth and the postnatal period. Consideration of this model in relation to the models developed by Rubin (1984) and Mercer (1986) suggests that combination of elements of these models may assist in the assessment of the needs of women at different stages in pregnancy and after the birth.

In using the Activities of Living Model, each activity is assessed in relation to the life-span, independence/dependence and the five influencing factors. The five influencing factors are grouped into three components: the physical or physiological, social–cultural and physiological, in descriptions of the assessment process (Roper *et al*, 1981; Pearson and Vaughan, 1986). Such an assessment can produce a detailed picture of the total needs of the childbearing woman, including psychological and educational needs, as shown by Taylor and Coventry (1983), a midwifery clinical teacher and student midwife. They provide an example of the application of the model in the care of a woman in the early postnatal period. This illustrates the contribution of the model to the identification of a range of potential and actual problems across the spectrum of activities of living. Trials of the model led to identification of social problems being experienced by one woman, causing her anxiety which had not been identified previously by the ward staff. This example illustrates the value of a framework on which to base an assessment, rather than practice based on no apparent framework, which may lead to problems being overlooked.

However, the assessment guidelines provided by Roper *et al.* (1981) do appear to focus on physical needs. Henderson (1990) has commented on this drawback of the model in relation to the childbearing woman: The model is excellent in relation to physical aspects of care. Social/educational aspects are referred to but do not seem to be as important, although during childbirth these areas, including the cultural aspects, are extremely relevant' (Henderson, 1990, p. 59).

This apparent drawback with the model may be a function of the way it has been applied, rather than being inherent in it. The need for assessment of socio-cultural factors is particularly important in pregnancy and childbirth, even in areas in which a physical assessment may be considered adequate. Wiedenbach (1967) provides an illustration of the need to assess socio-cultural factors as well as the physical in the description of a woman who was unable to meet her elimination needs: she had not had a spontaneous bowel-movement by the fourth postpartum day. The woman described how she had a bowel-movement just prior to the birth of her baby in the presence of her doctor:

> 'And there – when they had me up on the table – I could feel my bowels move with a strong contraction. I could have died on the spot. My doctor and a stranger stood right there at the foot of the table and saw me do it. A nurse was there too. I couldn't help myself and I couldn't hide. What must they have thought of me?' Tears rolled down her cheeks as she poured out the story. The nurse listened sympathetically and was understanding of Mrs T's embarrassment and distress. (Wiedenbach, 1967, p. 352)

It was explained to the woman that this act, which she saw as breaking socio-cultural taboos, was viewed by those present as a sign of good progress in labour rather than anything else. A straight physiological assessment would have resulted in her having another enema (according to the practice at that time), rather than the normal bowel-movement she was able to have following this discussion.

Nursing care described by the Activities of Living Model is based on the stages of the process of nursing, assessment, planning, implementation and evaluation (Roper *et al.* 1981; Aggleton and Chalmers, 1986). The model describes three types of activity which are undertaken by people to meet needs (or by nurses/midwives to implement care): preventing activities, comforting activities and seeking activities (Roper *et al.* 1983; Pearson and Vaughan, 1986). These activities may be carried out by the individual or by someone else, such as a midwife, on behalf of an individual depending on the need, the person's dependency and position in the life-span. Preventing activities are aimed at preventing ill health – for example, stopping smoking in pregnancy or having childhood immunisations. Comforting activities are aimed at reducing discomfort – for example, wearing comfortable clothes in pregnancy. Seeking activities are aimed at obtaining information – for example, attending antenatal classes or seeking care. Nursing activities are described by the model as comprising a preventing component, a comfort component and a dependent component. This last is derived from the seeking activities of the individual and appears to describe the activities of the nurse which are medically prescribed such as administration of medicines (Roper *et al.*, 1983, p. 9) (that is, that in certain areas of nursing practice nursing is dependent on medicine).

Application of this model requires assessment of the childbearing woman in relation to her position in the life-span, her dependence/ independence and needs in relation to the activities of living in terms of physical, socio-cultural and psychological aspects. Care to meet these needs is then identified in terms of the type of activity required to meet the need. The model is focused on the individual and their present abilities to maintain their health within the context of their physical, social and psychological needs.

McDonald (1986) provides an illustration of the use of the model in the care of a woman in labour and makes the point that the wide-ranging nature of the assessment makes it difficult to apply for the first time with a woman on admission in labour. She suggests that the model should be used during the care of the woman antenatally and gives support and health education as examples of needs that could have been addressed by the use of the model in the antenatal period. McDonald (1986) also highlights another problem in the use of this (or perhaps any other model) in childbearing: the presence of two people for whom care is being provided, the woman and her infant. Mercer (1986) has partly addressed this issue in her attention to the effect of the infant's health and other variables on the mother after birth; and the models of antenatal care consider the quality and nature of dyad relationships (mother–fetus/infant and mother–partner) and the factors which influence those relationships (Mercer *et al.*, 1988).

This discussion suggests that the Activities of Living Model has potential in the care of the childbearing woman and the results of surveys discussed earlier indicate that it is a model that is being widely used (Hughes and Goldstone, 1989; Murphy-Black, 1992a and b) although it is still the case, as McDonald commented in 1986, that there are few publications demonstrating or testing the use of this model in practice, in the care of the childbearing woman.

ROSEMARY METHVEN: APPLICATION OF OREM'S AND HENDERSON'S MODELS TO MIDWIFERY CARE

Rosemary Methven is a British midwife and midwife lecturer whose research and writing since the early 1980s has been concerned to counter the medical/obstetric focus of much midwifery practice and make explicit the needs of women for midwifery care (Methven, 1982; 1989; 1990). In the early 1980s she undertook a study of 40 women attending for antenatal booking at four hospitals (Methven, 1990b). The booking interviews were conducted by the antenatal clinic staff (midwives and student midwives) using the obstetric notes used at each hospital. Methven observed each interview, which was tape recorded, interviewed the staff who undertook the bookings and interviewed each of the women herself, using an assessment tool based on Orem's Self-Care Deficit Theory of Nursing.

Methven found that the booking interviews were conducted in a ritualistic manner which followed the structure of the obstetric record. Closed questions were used in the main, limiting discussion but also contributing to inaccuracies in the recorded information. Only three open questions occurred in the 40 interviews and Methven comments on possible reasons for lack of such questions:

> Pressure of time may have prevented more of these questions being asked, or it could have been that the obstetric notes did not provide space for this type of information to be recorded. It is also possible that the interviewing midwives were not interested in obtaining this sort of information about women, and did not view them holistically but rather as obstetric objects. (Methven, 1989, p. 53).

The midwives and student midwives, by their use of closed questions, limited interaction with the women. The topic headings on the obstetric record also limited that interaction to medical topics, including, for example, the past obstetric history and menstrual history, while aspects of the woman's care which might be described as midwifery concerns were either ignored or not raised at all:

> The result in terms of the content of the interview was a substantial amount of data concerning medical and obstetric history, but practically nothing about the woman's responses to childbirth, her feelings

concerning her present pregnancy, and her views on the management of her past or present confinement. (Methven, 1989, p. 58).

Methven concluded from these observations that the midwives were working within a medical model of care. This model was reinforced by the structure of the obstetric notes and the organisation of the hospital antenatal clinics. It is evident that the midwives included in this study had little or no responsibility for the care provided or for continuity of care, although several permanent clinic midwives emphasised the importance of the booking visit for establishing a relationship with the woman. Their care also reflects the attitudes held about them by obstetricians whom Methven approached when gaining access to undertake the study:

> The chairman, an obstetrician who only practised gynaecology, commented: 'The midwife plays such an insignificant part in the overall initial visit to clinic by mothers at this hospital, that I wonder if it is worthwhile doing a study on such a small part.' (Methven, 1989, p. 47)

Such an attitude is in marked contrast to the view of the first meeting between the pregnant woman and her midwife described by Davis (1987): 'This very personal, indepth meeting with the parents is your opportunity to understand their ideals surrounding birth and parenting, and to provide them with appropriate information' (p. 9).

Following the interview with the midwife, Methven interviewed each woman, using an assessment schedule based on the concept of universal self-care requisites which forms part of Orem's model. These assessments were then compared with the assessments made using the obstetric notes. The assessments provided a much more detailed picture of the individuality of the woman and her circumstances, her needs and expectations. In addition, the assessment provided greater information about 'medical' or obstetric' aspects of care – for example, use of contraception and diet (Methven, 1986a, 1989):

> But in every case she emerged as a person in her own right, with views and feelings about her baby, opinions about her care and management in pregnancy and labour. Her family, activities of daily living and her present physiological and psychological responses to pregnancy were also brought into focus. (Methven, 1989, p. 63)

Through this research, Methven has shown clearly the influence of the model of care on the care provided. The medical/obstetric model epitomised in the obstetric notes limited the midwives' attention, whereas the use of a nursing model enabled Methven to explore areas which were of concern to the women and important in holistic midwifery care.

Methven was concerned to understand the whole process of assessment, identification of needs and problems, implementation and evaluation of care relating to the childbearing woman; that is, the use of a needs/problem solving approach, the midwifery/nursing process. The booking interview is the beginning of the assessment phase of the nursing process and it is in this sense that Methven (1989) refers to 'the nursing process interview'. As discussed previously, the nursing process is a tool which enables systematic assessment, planning, implementation and evaluation. This tool may be used within any model of care and, indeed, has been widely used within the medical world in the form of problem-orientated medical records. While use of the nursing process may open up the idea that women have needs (something not acknowledged to any great extent by the midwives observed by Methven), it is the model within which the midwifery/nursing process is used which will give direction to the questioning and care provided. Methven undertook her research in the early 1980s and by 1990 she suggests, perhaps rather optimistically, that midwives' attitudes may have changed:

> It is assumed that you are already aware of the following....
>
> How to design a care plan using the nursing/midwifery process or planned individualised care based on a suitable framework or model of care. (Methven, 1990, pp. 42–3)

Methven applied a nursing model to midwifery practice as:

> A unique midwifery model may well be necessary and may come to fruition in the future, but none exists at present. It is therefore necessary to utilise a model that has already been tried, even though it was originally designed for use in general nursing. (Methven, 1986a, p. 16)

Orem first developed the model of self-care deficit in 1958 and has published several revisions of the theory since (Eben *et al.*, 1989). The central model draws on theory and knowledge in psychology and is based on six concepts: self-care; self-care capabilities (self-care agency); therapeutic self-care demand; self-care deficit; nursing agency; and nursing system. The central philosophy of the model is based on the view that people are able to undertake self-care for the majority of the time but may at times require help (when they have a self-care deficit) (Johnston, 1989, p. 165).

Self-care is comprised of three types of self-care requisites:

1. Universal self-care requisites. These are common to all human beings during all stages of the life cycle, and are adjusted according to age, developmental state, environment and other factors.
2. Developmental self-care requisites. These are associated with human developmental processes and conditions and events during various stages of the life cycle, for example, prematurity and pregnancy.
3. Health deviation self-care requisites. These are associated with genetic and constitutional defects and human structural-functional deviation, together with their effects, medical diagnosis and treatment. (Methven, 1986a, p. 15)

Orem describes eight universal self-care requisites and Methven (1986a; 1989) illustrates assessment of the requisites in the antenatal booking interview:

1. The maintenance of a sufficient intake of food, for example:

    1e. Has there been any alteration in your usual eating pattern since you became pregnant?
2. The maintenance of a sufficient intake of water, for example:

    2e. Do you know what fluid requirements are recommended when you are pregnant?
3. The provision of care associated with elimination processes and excrements, for example:

    5f. Do you usually pass urine without difficulty?
4. The maintenance of a sufficient intake of air, for example:

    4b. Do you know how breathing may be affected during pregnancy?
5. The maintenance of a balance between activity and rest, for example:

    3b. Do you pursue any sports or undertake any vigorous exercise?
6. The prevention of hazard to human life, human functioning and human wellbeing, for example:

    8g. Is there anything that usually makes you feel stressed or anxious?
7. The maintenance of a balance between solitude and social interaction, for example:

    9h. What is your reaction to being cared for by hospital staff and midwives whom you may not have met before?

8. The promotion of human functioning and development within social groups in accord with human potential, known human limitations and the human desire to be normal, for example:

6c. What have you read or what do you know about having a baby and becoming a mother? (Methven, 1989, pp. 51, 68, 69)

Self-care capabilities (agency) is the ability of the individual to meet their own needs or the needs of a dependant, such as a baby. The therapeutic self-care demand describes the need for help to maintain or promote health, and the self-care deficit describes the deficit between the therapeutic self-care demand and the ability of the individual to meet these demands through exercising self-care capabilities. The nursing agency acts to meet this deficit through one of three nursing systems: wholly compensatory, in which the nurse/midwife acts for the person who is unable to meet their own needs (for example, if unconscious or on bed-rest, postnatally experiencing side-effects of epidural anaesthesia); partly compensatory when the nurse/midwife undertakes some activities for the individual (for example, care activities in labour); and supportive-educative, where the individual is able to undertake self-care activities but needs assistance to do so (for example, a woman gaining confidence in breast-feeding (Eben *et al.*, 1989, p. 121).

Within the nursing system, five methods of assistance are described:

(i)   Acting or doing for another;
(ii) Guiding another;
(iii) Supporting another (physically or psychologically;
(iv) Providing an environment that promotes personal development in relation to becoming able to meet present or future demands for action;
(v)   Teaching another. (Methven, 1986a, p. 14)

The philosophy behind this approach to practice is that individuals are essentially self-caring and that it is the role of the nurse or midwife to identify self-care deficits and act in ways to either compensate for the individual's inability to meet their needs or support the individual in meeting their needs. A midwifery assessment would therefore include assessment and planning of care within the six concept areas. Methven has illustrated the use of this model in the care of a woman throughout the childbearing process (Methven, 1986a). In this illustration Methven concentrates on the assessment of universal self-care requisites, commenting that developmental self-care requisites have been assessed by the interview conducted using the obstetric notes, and that assessment of health-deviation self-care requisites is unnecessary 'for the purpose of the present study, which concentrates on a woman who expects to be in a state of normal health' (Methven, 1986a, p. 16).

Developmental self-care requisites relate to the process of maturation (Eben *et al.*, 1989) and in terms of childbearing relate to the role-change which is central to the model of maternal role development proposed and tested by Rubin (1984). It is possible that incorporation of some of the concepts from Rubin's model would enhance the understanding of the meaning of developmental self-care requisites in pregnancy.

In a similar way, incorporation of an understanding of potential health deviations in the childbearing process, which are central to an obstetric history, might assist in the assessment of health deviation self-care requisites. Methven has demonstrated that use of this model assists the identification of women's social, psychological and physical needs but, due to the circumstances of her research, this assessment had to be tacked on to the obstetric history taking. An assessment process constructed around the use of Orem's model which incorporates elements from the obstetric/medical history into assessment of health deviation self-care requisites would provide the vital obstetric/medical information while at the same time enabling the woman's individual concerns to be identified, and form a basis for individual care throughout her pregnancy within a system of midwifery-led care.

Methven (1986b) has also provided a description of the use of Virginia Henderson's approach to nursing in the care of a woman during the childbirth process. It is not surprising that Methven considers that both Henderson and Orem provide a framework or model which can be used in the care of the childbearing woman, as the two approaches are very similar.

Henderson (1969) has defined nursing as follows:

> The unique function of the nurse is to assist the individual, sick or well, in the performance of those activities contributing to health or its recovery (or to a peaceful death) that he would perform unaided if he had the necessary strength, will or knowledge. And to do this in such a way as to help him gain independence as rapidly as possible. (Henderson, 1969, p. 4)

The assistance of the nurse is focused on 14 basic needs or activities of daily living (Methven, 1986b; De Neester *et al.*, 1989). Eben *et al.* (1989) identify Henderson as one of the people who influenced Orem in her theory development. The assisting role of the nurse in helping the person regain independence in activities of daily living has many similarities to the focus of the nursing agency on helping the person to achieve self-care through attention to self-care deficits. Runk and Quillin (1989) comment that Henderson did not describe her definition as a theory, but the concepts within the definition can be analysed and seen to form the basis of a model.

Another interesting feature of Henderson's definition is its focus on health and education. Although in the world of the illness-nurse this aspect may not have been emphasised, if the definition is slightly re-arranged it can be seen more clearly to apply to the work of the health-nurse in the community and to the midwife:

> The unique function of the *midwife* is to assist the woman, *well* or sick, in the performance of those activities contributing to *health* or its recovery (or to a peaceful death) that she would perform unaided if she had the necessary knowledge, will or strength. And to do this in such a way as to help her gain independence as rapidly as possible.

Methven (1986b) discusses the contribution that Henderson's model made to care and also the difficulties in applying the model. Through her work with Orem and Henderson's models, Methven was one of the initiators of the practical work and theoretical discussion which is needed to understand the way midwives think about how care influences the care provided. Methven is concerned to make the elements and concepts of midwifery practice explicit to enable midwives to identify the wide needs that women have and to make explicit the midwifery care needed to meet these needs. Lack of a midwifery model led her to explore the relevance of nursing models for midwifery but she concludes at the end of her discussion of the use of Henderson's model:

> As such her 'model' may be said to be an improvement on the practice of performing midwifery assessment which is not based on any framework other than tradition. However, a model satisfactorily designed for midwifery, based on health and not on illness, resulting from research into what information midwives really need in order to provide effective care for the mother, and enabling the midwife to exercise her independent practitioner role within the health care team, has yet to be developed. (Methven, 1986b, p. 53)

THE ROY ADAPTATION MODEL

The Adaptation Model, initially developed by Sister Callista Roy in the 1960s, is another example of a grand nursing model developed from the knowledge base of theoretical and experimental psychology. This model has been used extensively in nursing practice, education and research and has also been used in the care of women during childbearing. Castledine and Jones (1987) provide an illustration of the use of this model in the care of the childbearing woman, while Fawcett and Tulman (1990) and Lynam and Miller (1991) have undertaken research into the relevance of the concepts included in the model to care of women during pregnancy.

The basis of the model is the view that people are biopsychosocial beings in constant interaction with their environment (Rambo, 1984). Generally the individual is able to manage this interaction and maintain their health but when there is a breakdown in the individual's ability to meet the demands of this interaction nursing, or midwifery, care will be required. The model includes three types of stimuli which affect the individual, their adaptation and thus health (Rambo, 1984; Aggleton and Chalmers, 1986; Pearson and Vaughan, 1986).

Focal stimuli are found in the immediate environment and are the main factors which influence the person – for example, the health or ill-health of the newly-born baby will have an immediate effect on the health of the new mother. Contextual stimuli are the general factors which surround the woman. For example, poor living conditions and the extent of family support will affect the extent to which she is able to cope with (adapt to) ill-health in her child. Residual stimuli are internal factors which are personal to the individual, their beliefs, experiences and attitudes. For example, if the woman has had a poor experience of maternity care in the past she will bring this experience to her expectations of future care.

These stimuli are described as affecting the individual in four areas or modes of their lives: the physiological mode, the self-concept mode, the role function mode and the interdependence mode. The physiological mode is concerned with the functioning of the body, and needs emerge when there is disruption in the physiological processes of:

Oxygenation and circulation
Fluid and electrolyte balance
Nutrition
Elimination
Rest and activity

Regulation: temperature, sensory, and hormonal (Rambo, 1984, pp. 11–12)

The self-concept mode is concerned with the individual's view of themselves. Rambo (1984) describes this concept as having two aspects. The first relates to concern with the body: what am I? The second relates to the self: who am I? The concern with the body relates to body-functioning and body-image and may be an issue of particular concern during pregnancy and following childbirth. The second concern is with consistency of the self-image: 'The personal self is concerned with self-consistency, self-ideal, and the moral-ethical self as one seeks to cope with getting to know oneself.' (Rambo, 1984, p. 12) and again this aspect of the self is changing and developing during childbearing.

The role function mode is concerned with the extent to which the individual is able to respond to the demands and expectations from society and themselves in the performance of their roles. This mode is the central concern of the work of Rubin (1984) and others discussed in Chapter 6.

The interdependence mode describes the balance that people seek to achieve between independence and dependence on others. Aggleton and Chalmers (1986) comment that when people are placed in situations outside their normal experience (there is a change in the contextual variables) they may react with aggression or feel alienation or loneliness, which will affect their behaviour. Midwifery care would then be aimed at ameliorating the contextual variables that threaten the person's interdependence – for example, on admission to a labour ward.

Also included in the model is the concept of limited energy. People are described, on the life continuum and the health–illness continuum, as having different levels of energy and thus different abilities to respond to the demands of the focal, contextual and residual stimuli, and meet their physiological, self-concept, role function and interdependence needs (Rambo, 1984; Aggleton and Chalmers, 1986).

Using the approach of assessment, problem identification, mutual goal-setting, intervention and evaluation needs are assessed, in relation to these modes and the extent to which focal, contextual and residual stimuli are inhibiting the individual's ability to adapt to the stimulus (Fawcett, 1984). First-level assessment describes the individual's behaviour, and second-level assessment describes the stimuli which have affected the person's behaviour or adaptation (Pearson and Vaughan, 1986). Midwifery action is aimed at identifying needs in relation to the four modes and the three stimuli and supporting the women in interventions either to modify the stimuli, if this is possible, in developing the woman's energy, or supporting the woman in other ways in the process of adaptation and maintenance of her health.

The Adaptation Model takes a holistic approach to assessment and care and, while it includes attention to physiological factors, three of the modes are concerned with what might generally be termed psychosocial areas: self-concept, role functioning and interdependence. Castledine and Jones (1987) describe their interest in the application of the Roy Adaptation Model in midwifery as arising from a review of midwifery records which showed little recording of psychosocial information by midwives. They describe the use of an assessment schedule in the antenatal period, which included assessment of intrapersonal factors (self-concept mode), interpersonal factors (role function mode), interdependency mode factors and physical examination (physiological mode).

Areas assessed under the self-concept mode included moods and feelings, body image, sexuality, methods of coping and pain assessment. The assessment of the role function mode included assessment of the roles held by the woman, and any conflict between different roles and the adoption of new roles:

> This area covers the patient's usual role and changing role functions and relationships with others either as a pregnant woman or as a mother in relation to others at home or at work. It surprises many when their role is split in two, i.e. of a wife and a mother. (Castledine and Jones, 1987, p. 8)

Factors assessed in the interdependence mode include the extent to which the woman is dependent on her family and on health care practitioners such as the midwife and the general practitioner. This example provides an early illustration of the use of the Roy Adaptation Model in midwifery. As discussed above, this model is now quite widely used in midwifery care in Britain (Hughes and Goldstone, 1989; Murphy-Black, 1992a). Castledine and Jones (1987) comment that the model has altered midwifery practice by helping midwives to be more aware of psychosocial needs and has helped women feel more involved in their care.

This model was developed by Roy deductively from existing theory and there is a need to test the relationships hypothesised in the model through research (Tiedeman, 1989). Interestingly there are a number of studies by American researchers in the field of maternity care which have sought to test aspects of the model. Lynam and Miller (1991) describe a study of the extent to which there is agreement between women experiencing preterm labour and nurses caring for them, about their needs in the four modes. A sample of women (following birth) and a sample of nurses completed a questionnaire which asked them to rank 56 statements of needs in order of importance. Statements were devised which related to needs in each of the four modes.

The results showed statistically significant differences between the order in which the needs were ranked by the two groups. The women gave greater priority to the following needs than the nurses: 'To be asked opinions and preferences regarding type of delivery (self-concept mode)' and 'To be assured of a safe outcome for my baby (interdependence mode)'(Lynam and Miller, 1991, p. 133). In contrast, the nurses gave greater importance to protecting the women's privacy than the women gave to this need themselves. Both groups rated self-concept needs as being the most important for this group of women who had experienced preterm labour. The authors acknowledge the limitations of their study but conclude that the use of the Roy Adaptation Model may be useful with this group of women. The model helps to focus care on psychosocial needs, which are of greatest concern to women. The authors suggest that the psychosocial needs of this group of women may have received less attention, as the focus of care would be on the physical need to inhibit the progress of preterm labour.

Jacqueline Fawcett provides another illustration of the testing of the Roy Adaptation Model in care of the childbearing woman. Fawcett, a nurse theorist, has developed a programme of research which is aimed at testing the role function mode in the model. This programme of research began with a study which developed a tool which could be used in subsequent studies to measure the woman's role function at different times following childbirth. This tool was used to assess whether there were any differences in role functioning between women who had had normal deliveries, compared to those who had had Caesarean sections. The focal stimulus is the type of birth, and data were collected about this, using a record sheet. The contextual stimuli measured include demographic and health variables. Data relating to the role function mode were then analysed in relation to the information collected relating to the stimuli. Other tools have been developed as part of this research programme and further studies undertaken.

Two articles which form part of this programme of research derived from the Roy model, report the findings of a study of preparation of women during the antenatal period for Caesarean section (Fawcett, 1990; Fawcett *et al.*, 1993). Early studies showed that women had problems in all four adaptation areas after unplanned Caesarean sections, the focal stimulus. A nurse-midwifery intervention was therefore developed to ameliorate the effects of these unplanned operations, through attention to contextual stimuli, by making information about Caesarean sections available to women prior to labour. A leaflet was designed and group sessions were held during antenatal classes at which Caesarean section was discussed. These interventions were tested by a number of studies and this was followed by an experimental study. The experimental study was undertaken to test three hypotheses, which are summarised as follows: 'The hypotheses were based on the Roy Adaptation Model proposition that management of contextual stimuli promotes adaptation.' (Fawcett *et al.*, 1993, p. 52).

The study was undertaken with a control group, of women having planned Caesarean sections who had no intervention; an experimental group, comprising women who had unplanned Caesarean sections and normal deliveries who received the intervention: the class and the leaflet developed in earlier studies about Caesarean sections, in the antenatal course; and a control group of women who followed an antenatal class but did not have any additional input on Caesarean sections. The four modes were tested in the study using a number of measurement tools, including a pain measurement tool which measured aspects of the physiological mode and a self-esteem inventory which measured aspects of the self-concept mode.

The study found no correlations between the intervention and the hypotheses. A range of explanations suggest reasons for this lack of relationship, including changes in obstetric care since the start of the research programme, with the use of regional anaesthesia reducing the effects of unplanned Caesarean sections and the length of time between the intervention and the measurement of the outcomes. While this research was not able to demonstrate any relationship between variables in the model (adaptation and attention to contextual variables) it does demonstrate the potential of testing the model in care of the childbearing woman. The lack of relationship in this case, in addition, raises questions about the effects of antenatal classes on learning and behaviours postnatally and suggests a need to find additional ways of supplying information. This research also has similarities to the research by Hayward (1975) on information-giving prior to surgery, which would perhaps add support to the view that the information has to be given closer to the event to influence adaptation.

NEUMAN SYSTEMS MODEL

Spires (1991) argues that the Neuman Systems Model, developed by Betty Neuman, is useful in midwifery practice, as the model takes as its starting-point the well individual or well community. The person or community, termed the client system, is depicted as a central, energy core surrounded by lines of resistance and the normal line of defence. The central core comprises physiological, psychological, sociocultural, developmental and spiritual variables. The lines of resistance illustrate the ability of the client system to maintain its state of equilibrium. The normal line of defence demonstrates the usual state of health of the person and provides a standard against which deviations in health can be measured (Neuman, 1989). The normal line of defence is threatened by stressors in the environment in which the individual is located. Three types of environment are identified: the external environment, which includes interpersonal relationships; the internal environment, which consists of intrapersonal forces occurring within the client system; and the created-environment, which is subconsciously created and which 'goes beyond the internal and external environments encompassing both'(Neuman, 1989, p. 32).

While this description of the model hints at the more abstruse aspects of some of the nursing models, the three environments are generally labelled as intrapersonal, interpersonal and extrapersonal. Assessment is concerned with identifying the effects of stressors in any of these environments on the five groups of variables. Intervention is then aimed at reinforcing the line of defence and increasing the ability of the system, the individual, to cope with the stressor which is impinging on the defence line protecting the system. A further element in this model is the inclusion of primary, secondary and tertiary prevention activities which are aimed at ameliorating the effects of stressors. The inclusion of these concepts reinforces the preventive and health promotive approach to care which is implicit in this model, which Spires (1991) identifies as its value for midwifery practice:

> In this model, then, childbirth is perceived to be a normal process. The midwife's role lies mainly in primary prevention, to strengthen the mother–fetus internal lines of resistance and outer lines of defence to enable them to cope with stressors and prevent the need for medical intervention. (Spires, 1991, p. 10)

In her discussion of the model, Spires (1991) provides examples of intrapersonal, interpersonal and extrapersonal factors and these are further illustrated by Dunn and Trépanier (1989) in a discussion of the Neuman Systems Model in perinatal care. Considering the woman and the fetus as one unit, they identify the following examples of sources of intrapersonal stress affecting the five groups of variables:

Physiological:	Maternal – weight gain, incompetent cervix; Fetus – hypoxia, genetic problems
Psychological:	Anxiety, grief process
Sociocultural:	Role conflict, cultural beliefs
Developmental:	Educational level, developmental tasks of pregnancy
Spiritual:	Beliefs affecting pregnancy and childbirth (Dunn and Trépanier, 1989, p. 414)

These examples illustrate the utility of the model in the care of the childbearing woman and the incorporation in the model of a large range of concepts and variables which need to be considered by the midwife if the wellbeing of the woman and fetus/infant is to be optimised.

RIEHL'S INTERACTIONIST MODEL OF NURSING

Neuman's model, discussed above, is based on systems theory and the individual is described as a system in interaction with the surrounding and internal environments. In contrast, the model developed by Riehl is concerned with the meanings that people ascribe to situations:

> According to this alternative perspective, people behave as they do, not because of the workings of systems within them, but because of meanings attached to the actions they perform. (Aggleton and Chalmers, 1986, p. 71)

This model is based on the theories developed by symbolic interactionists, as are the models developed by Rubin (1984) and Mercer (1986), discussed in Chapter 6. Riehl describes three aspects or parameters of behaviour: physiological, psychological and sociological parameters. Individuals strive to make sense of their world and when there is a disturbance in one or more parameters, for example during pregnancy, the individual makes attempts to redefine or understand the situation (Aggleton and Chalmers, 1986).

Roach and Brown (1991) describe the adoption of this model in a group of London hospitals. The model was chosen, in part, because of its focus on the psychological rather than the physical needs of the woman. In addition, the model emphasises the need for the midwife to make a relationship with the woman, to enter into her world and to help the woman with the development of new roles. This process involves role-taking, which is described by Aggleton and Chalmers (1986) as 'primarily involving thinking about a situation from another's point of view' (p. 78). Both the midwife and the woman may undertake this activity to increase their understanding of the situation, to see the situation in different ways and to test out new roles (Aggleton and Chalmers, 1986, p. 78).

Aggleton and Chalmers (1986) illustrate their discussion of this model with reference to midwifery care, and suggest that the midwife who puts herself in the position of the woman is better able to appreciate the demands on the woman and to help her cope with the demands of the role of mother. This role-taking, they suggest, may also help to modify the expectations of the midwife and lead to compromise between the aims of the midwife and the type of care that the woman is providing to her baby. This role-taking is a particular feature of Riehl's model and implies a close relationship between the woman and the midwife. It may be for this reason that Roach and Brown (1991) conclude that this model may be more easily adopted in a situation where team midwifery is practised.

DEVELOPMENT OF LOCAL AND OTHER MODELS

Descriptions of the development of models in practice are rather sparse in the literature but Telfer (1991) and Carter (1992) provide evidence that local model development may be taking place which has not yet been reported in the literature. The models discussed here all have a common starting-point in the view of their developers: that nursing models did not encompass the whole of midwifery care, or laid the emphasis of care on certain aspects, such as physical care or activities of living which, while important, were of lesser concern in care of women who were essentially healthy than in care of the person with an illness (Mayes, 1987; Henderson, 1990; Smith, 1991).

Henderson (1990) describes the gradual development of the Human Needs Model for Midwifery in one maternity unit over a period of four years. This development started with the introduction of birth plans, identification of the unit philosophy, recognition of the need for a model to guide practice, review of current models, development of a model and testing of the model in practice. Seven benefits of using a model for midwifery are suggested:

It coordinates the beliefs of midwives about the care they give.
It enables continuity of care.
It furthers the giving of consistent advice.
It improves record-keeping.
It assists in the identification of poor practice.
It aids the development of research into midwifery practice.
It supports the practitioner's autonomy. (Henderson, 1990, p. 60)

This model considers the four areas which are the key aspects of any model: the person (or in this case persons, the woman, her baby and family); health; the environment or context for care; and midwifery practice. The Human Needs Model for Midwifery is based, in addition, on the work of Minshull *et al.* (1986). These nurse educators developed the Human Needs Model of Nursing, following extensive discussions in one health authority, with the aim of developing a model which was relevant to British nursing and which it was possible to apply in nursing practice, education and research. One of the concerns of these authors was that many nursing models concentrate on the individual's physical needs while much nursing practice is with well individuals, a sentiment with which many midwives will have sympathy. Minshull *et al.* (1986), for example, calculate that 58 per cent of the nursing activities identified by Roper *et al.* (1983) are orientated towards meeting physical needs.

The Human Needs Model for nursing is based on Maslow's hierarchy of human need which suggests that individuals have different types of needs: physical needs; safety and security needs; needs for love and belongingness; self-esteem and dignity needs and self-actualisation needs. While there is an implication in the model that lower-order needs should be met before the person can pay attention to higher-order needs, Minshull *et al.* (1986) reject this and suggest that nursing care should be directed at needs within all the first four levels. Interestingly, they suggest that self-actualisation needs can be only met by individuals themselves but that nursing activity to meet needs in other areas can enable individuals to meet their self-actualisation needs.

Self-actualisation is described as 'the individual reaching their full potential' (Minshull *et al.*, 1986, p. 646). If pregnancy and childbirth are seen as times of role change and growth, it can be argued that women are seeking to meet their needs at this level and it may be that midwifery care should be directed at assisting in this process as well as assisting with meeting needs at the other levels.

In Henderson's (1990) Human Needs Model for Midwifery the four areas of need are designated as physical needs; social needs; psychological needs; and educational needs. Using this model throughout the process of childbearing, with the process of assessment, planning, implementation and evaluation, midwifery care is orientated towards helping to meet the physical, social, psychological and educational needs of the woman, her partner, her baby and wider family. The midwife and woman are described as working as partners in care which aims to meet individual needs and which acknowledges the altered state of health that pregnancy represents rather than seeing pregnancy as a state of ill-health (Henderson, 1990). The hierarchy of need appears to be accepted in this model:

> The categories of need are based on Maslow's hierarchy of human needs and emphasise that to maintain health in the mother and baby a sequence of need should be followed. A foundation of physical well-being should be laid before psychological, spiritual, social and finally educational well-being can be achieved. (Henderson, 1990, p. 62)

The meeting of needs in a hierarchical manner may not be borne out in practice, as Henderson (1986) illustrates with a practice example. This illustration shows the concurrent existence of needs at the different levels in the care of a woman in the early postnatal period.

In an unpublished model for midwifery care, A Framework for Midwifery Care Contingent on Need, cultural needs as well as physical, psychological, educational and social needs are addressed (Telfer, 1991). Carter (1992) proposes a philosophy of care, also unpublished (see Chapter 5) which should be read with this model. The focus of the model is the mother and baby, and individualised midwifery care is achieved through the use of the cycle of assessment, planning, imple-mentation, recording and evaluating care. Recording is highlighted as a separate activity, and the importance of recording is also addressed by Henderson (1990) who describes the revision of documentation which took place in a maternity unit with adoption of the Human Needs Model for Midwifery.

Additional elements in the model described by Telfer (1991) are the understanding and personal attributes that the midwife brings to the care of the childbearing woman. The attributes are described using the Five C's of Caring: compassion, competence, confidence, con-science and commitment, which have been incorporated from the work of Roach (1987). The model has its origins in a research study on the educational needs of young pregnant women (Telfer, 1990). The social and financial deprivation of some of the respondents was considerable, as was the obvious anxiety of those women who had suffered a previ-ous early pregnancy loss. Without understanding the implications of these matters for the individual woman and internalisation of the Five C's of caring, particularly compassion, Telfer (1993) argues that the individual needs of these women could not be understood and met. It is clear that the concept of caring is a significant concept for the further development of models for midwifery (Roach, 1987). As discussed in earlier parts of this book, the person of the midwife, the skills of the midwife and the knowledge of the midwife have a significant impact on the care provided, and inclusion of these concepts in models for midwifery would appear to be an essential, though rarely acknowledged, part of any model for midwifery care.

Midwives in Waltham Forest provide another illustration of the process of developing a model to guide practice (Mayes, 1987). The development of this model stemmed from the experience at the hospital of providing midwifery-led care in a short-stay unit, coupled with the process of developing a new midwifery curriculum. Collection of audit data showed care provided in the midwifery-led unit as compared to care in the main labour ward involved less intervention. The midwives identified together the principles, or concepts, which were incorporated into their model of care, and Mayes (1987) comments: 'it was interesting to note the consistency and clarity of their beliefs' (pp. vii–ix). Mayes (1987) defines and describes the principles of the model:

1 Childbirth is viewed as a normal, if major, life-event and the midwife's role is identified as assisting the woman to adapt to the stresses imposed by pregnancy and childbirth.

2 Each woman is identified as a unique individual with social, psychological, physical and cultural needs and expectations of childbearing: 'Such expectations include a safe confinement, a healthy baby, successful social relationships through the family, and above all, a personal sense of independence and self fulfilment.' (Mayes, 1987, p. vi). These aims are very similar, although expressed in different terms, to the maternal tasks of pregnancy identified by Rubin (1984) and discussed in Chapter 6. This model identifies the rights of the woman to informed choice; professional, competent support and autonomy in making decisions about her own care.

3 Communication: the principle of communication is seen as fundamental to the model on which the individualised care described above will be based. Without adequate communication the rights of the woman cannot be met.

4 Midwifery is described as being holistic. This term encompasses the wide range of needs of the individual woman, the diversity of cultural backgrounds and the need for midwives to be concerned with wider issues: 'The need to recognise social and cultural disadvantages and inequalities in health and maternity care was identified, in order that women may be helped to exercise their rights to fulfil their needs.' (Mayes, 1987, p. vii)

5 Midwifery care is provided in a planned, systematic manner. The care that is provided through assessment, planning, implementation and evaluation is based on the above principles so that at all stages the woman's autonomy is protected, her individual needs are addressed and so forth.

Two additional principles are identified: the need for a research base for practice, and the characterisation of midwifery care as comprising two parts: health promotion and clinical care. This neat differentiation helps to get round the frequent difficulty that midwives express in relation to the use of the term 'problem' in relation to midwifery care with women who are essentially healthy. The systematic approach is illustrated as two circles. The outer circle is concerned with the identification of health needs, the provision of support to meet these needs and the evaluation: 'Has health been maintained?' (Mayes, 1987, p. vii). The inner circle is concerned with the identification of problems and the provision of clinical midwifery care to meet those problems.

The identification of these principles provides a clear framework for practice and, if they were described in measurable terms, it would be possible to assess to what extent these concepts were being translated into practice.

The Newbourne model developed by a group of midwives in Hertfordshire provides another illustration of the development of a local model. Having examined and rejected a number of nursing models this group identified a number of concepts which led them to describe the process of development of the model as a process of discovery of commonly-held views: 'it seemed that the ideas expressed in the model have always been in the back of midwives' minds.' (Smith, 1991, p. 56). Midwifery care is described as holistic care and the focus of that care is the client pair: the mother and fetus or mother and baby.

The woman and baby are described as being affected by a number of factors: genes, physiological processes, feelings and experiences. The woman and baby are situated in an immediate and extended family within the context of a culture, beliefs and values and within the wider society and environment, which are additional factors which will have an influence on the woman and fetus/baby. During pregnancy, Smith (1991) describes the woman as going on a journey of change 'into a new state of life' (p. 57) and the midwife is her companion on this journey. The role of the midwife within this model is to identify any actual or potential problems in the woman's immediate and wider environment which may inhibit this journey:

> The midwife's goal, as her client makes her transition to mother-hood, is for the mother and fetus/baby to be normal and healthy, for the woman to feel confident and happy with her pregnancy and confinement, and to be supported by loving family and friends. She hopes that any conflicts which have arisen regarding her patient's culture will have been resolved and that the demands of society will have been met. (Smith, 1991, p. 57)

This model takes as its central concern the transition to motherhood which is central to some of the models considered in Chapter 6. To avoid the imposition on the woman of a great deal of questioning during the assessment process the women are given a care plan to complete. The areas assessed in the care plan relate to the factors which the model identifies as influencing the mother and fetus/baby, asking for example: 'Have you had any experiences which might help or trouble you as you approach motherhood this time?' (Smith, 1991, p. 58). This reinforces the concept of participation which runs through this model and contributes to the process of identifying a need for midwifery assistance which has echoes of Wiedenbach's (1967) need-for-help (see Chapter 6).

These examples all provide descriptions of the development of models by groups of midwives to guide practice in maternity units and across hospital and community care. In contrast, the model described by Littlewood (1989) may be seen as a more theoretical approach to model development which is largely informed by the research findings rather than the personal belief systems of groups of midwives. However, this model shares with those above a focus on the individual woman and concern with her needs. Littlewood (1989) describes the need to consider the signs of ill-health and the process of hospitalisation from the perspective of the woman herself and the meanings she may give to certain aspects of her health and care which will be determined by her cultural background.

Using the care of a woman admitted with pre-eclampsia Littlewood (1989) discusses the social meaning of the hospital and the need for the nurse (midwife) to be aware of the medical model and lay interpretations of the woman's health. Using this anthropological perspective of ascribed meaning the process of assessment, planning, implementation and evaluation of care carried out by the midwife will be concerned with the meaning ascribed as well as the woman's actual experience of signs and symptoms. Littlewood (1989) suggests that the adoption of an anthropological perspective may enable care to really move from being centred on tasks to being centred on the individual woman. Individualised care is an element of the models above but Littlewood (1989) helps to clarify one facet of individualised care and illustrates what is actually involved in achieving this type of care. This model is discussed further in relation to achieving participation in care in Chapter 4.

QUALITY ASSURANCE DEVELOPMENT

It may be suggested that all the work on the understanding and exploration of models of midwifery care is essentially concerned with the quality of care that the childbearing woman may experience from maternity services. In recent years there has been considerable activity in relation to the measurement of the quality of services, as Ball and Hughes (1993) discuss. This concern can be seen to be supported by the Health for All Model and the concept of affordable, effective, well-managed services (see Chapter 4). Review of the quality of services starts with an examination of the philosophies and goals of a service (which should, of course, also reflect the perceptions or definitions of the situation held by the consumers of that service, in this case the childbearing woman and her family). This is followed by measurement, for example the collection of information about the extent to which women are involved in their care, and comparison of the findings with the goals. Action is then taken, if necessary, to make changes to better meet the aims of the service.

The identification of ward, unit and national philosophies is a first step in this process (see Chapter 5). The care, the action, provided by a midwifery team will reflect their philosophy of care, as has been discussed earlier. The process of quality assurance involves examination of all aspects of the organisation and seeks to support alterations in any part of the organisation that is in need of change. The process of quality assurance therefore requires the clarification of values, models and theories of care and discussion between different occupational groups of their different models. The process of quality assurance and identification of the underlying models and theories held by midwives can thus be seen to be mutually reinforcing – activities in one area will support developments in the other.

Summary

This chapter began with a discussion of the use of the midwifery/ nursing process. It was argued that this is a tool which is incorporated into nursing models and assists in the application of these models in practice. An overview has been given of the work that has been undertaken (and is available) on the application of nursing models to midwifery and the development of local models. This discussion has shown that a range of models have the potential to clarify midwifery care and to help in the process of describing that care. It is clear, however, that a great deal of further work is required on testing these theories and models in practice. This discussion has been largely about deductive theories and their use in midwifery practice. It is interesting that the development of inductive theories (apart from those which may be identified in research findings, for example Kirkham (1989)) has been limited. It may be argued that these models do not reflect or expose the essence or concepts of midwifery care and do not use a language which describes that care. Kirkham (1989) has argued for the identification of these concepts. The models described in this chapter perhaps provide guidance but should be combined with additional observation and research to enable the construction of practice-based theories of midwifery.

Activities

Use these activities to reflect on this chapter and your own care.

1 Examine some care plans that you have written recently. What types of needs and problems predominate in the care plans? Do the needs and problems identified reflect your model or theories of midwifery?
2 What are the consequences of standard care plans for the woman's choice and control of her care?
3 Describe the contribution of any nursing models you have used in care of the childbearing woman. How did use of these models assist you in your care? What consequences did the model(s) have for the care experienced by childbearing women?
4 Is a model in use in the place in which you work? Describe the model in use and consider your views about the application of one conceptual model to care of all childbearing women.
5 Describe the differences in care that a woman might experience if care was provided using the Activities of Living Model, Orem's Self-Care Model and the Roy Adaptation Model.
6 Examine the way that women are booked for care where you are working. What model or models of care can you identify in this process? What are the consequences of this model or models on the actions (the care by the midwife) and the type of care experienced by the women?
7 How do the models described in this chapter relate to your personal model of midwifery care?
8 If you were developing a model for your practice, how would you go about this?

CHAPTER EIGHT

Developing theory for midwifery practice

That care should not be given in an erratic and whimsical way is not in dispute. Midwives do need to be sure of their role, what they have to offer women and to be able to approach individual women in a clear and thought out way. (Hughes, 1988, p. 3)

INTRODUCTION

The purpose of this book has been to present and discuss information which may contribute to the better understanding of the concepts, theories and models which inform midwifery practice. The increased understanding, achieved through clarification of concepts, theories and models, may then enable the further development of midwifery care in a context in which individual meanings and shared meanings have been made apparent. Discussion of concepts, theories and models either held or developed by midwives and nurse-midwives provides a basis for the further development or elucidation of those concepts, theories and models which are held by each midwife, each childbearing woman and by other health care practitioners involved in the provision of maternity care. While it is important, as referred to many times during the preceding chapters, for individual midwives to identify and describe their individual concepts of care, the context of midwifery care, discussed in Chapter 3, must always be remembered. The context has a significant effect on practice and there is a need to consider the concepts, theories and models held by midwives with those in society, in the organisation, held by those with whom midwives work and by the childbearing woman and her family.

In this final chapter the aim is to discuss a number of approaches to the process of identifying concepts, building and testing theories and moving towards the development of models of midwifery care. The preceding chapters have shown that there are basically two approaches to the process of identifying concepts, theories and models: the deductive and the inductive approaches which are considered below.

In Chapter 2 the idea of paradigms or world-views of knowledge was discussed. Although there may be discussions about the existence of such world-views in nursing (Robinson, 1992), Vaughan (1992) argues that there are three main world-views which inform the practice of nursing. These are the positivistic approaches of the natural sciences, the interpretative approaches of naturalism (that is, the study of the world from the perspective of those in the world and interpretation of their interactions) and critical social theory, a paradigm which contends that knowledge is based in practice which is explored through reflection and which seeks to liberate the thinking of the practitioner from the constraints of their personal social and historical context. The use of deductive theory is largely associated with the natural science paradigm, while interpretative approaches rest on the use of inductive methods and theorising. Critical social theory, of its very nature, is also an inductive approach to theory-generation. In the following discussion these three paradigms which, it may also be suggested, inform midwifery practice, will be considered. The first section, on deductive theory, is concerned with theory generated from a natural science perspective, while the second section, on inductive theory, considers both theory generated within the naturalism and critical social theory paradigms.

DEDUCTIVE APPROACHES

The identification of concepts and theories using the deductive approach involves examination of pre-existing knowledge or theory which is then applied to the practice of midwifery. This knowledge and theory may be part of the knowledge base of other disciplines, such as psychology; it may be found in models or theories of nursing, or it may be found in the literature about and on midwifery.

Use of theory from other disciplines

The use of theory from other disciplines is evident in a number of the theoretical developments discussed in earlier chapters. For example, at the beginning of Chapter 4 a number of disciplines and theories which have informed midwifery care were identified. These include physiological theories, for example about the process of breast-feeding; and sociological theories of postnatal depression; sociological theories, including change theory and systems theory, which contribute to the understanding of organisations; educational theories of adult learning which contribute to effective antenatal education; and many others.

In fact it is clear that midwifery practice could not continue if this knowledge base and theory developed in other fields was not used. As Price and Price (1993) comment:

> We, like the medical profession, should be comfortable in drawing on theory from other domains, such as physiology, pharmacology, psychology or sociology. Such theory helps us to anticipate, interpret and react to the changes in a woman's health status during pregnancy and beyond. (Price and Price, 1993, p. 235)

One approach to understanding theory and the concepts underpinning midwifery practice is, then, to identify the disciplines that inform midwifery care, to examine the concepts within those disciplines and their relevance to midwifery practice. This process, of concept clarification in these underlying disciplines, is found, for example, in textbooks on midwifery (Bennett and Brown, 1993; Silverton, 1993). Taking the example of labour, Silverton (1993) describes the need to understand the anatomy of the pelvis, the mechanism of muscle contraction and the physiology of uterine contractions, the mechanisms of labour, which include an understanding of the anatomy of the fetal skull, and the physiology of the separation of the placenta. An understanding of these concepts and the interrelationships between the concepts (theories about the concepts) contributes to the understanding of the process and mechanisms of labour.

This knowledge and theory appears quite straightforward and unproblematic but the way this knowledge is put into practice is where the personal concepts, theories and models of the midwife come into operation and where midwives may find cor.flict between their own models and those of the organisation or those of other health care practitioners (Field, 1983). Planning of labour care may involve establishing an atmosphere of mutual trust, using a birth plan (Silverton, 1993) but it also must take account of the local facilities (Silverton, 1993), hospital policies (which form the interpretation of theory) and the model of care supported by the organisation. Concepts and theory in this sense are not value-free. While the physiology of labour may be complex, it can be understood by the research scientist, the childbearing woman and the new student midwife on different levels, but the interpretation of that physiological process will vary from place to place. Interpretations may emphasise the waiting and watching approach, epitomised in the pregnancy as a normal life-event, or a more active, interventionist approach may be taken to the physiology of childbirth (Rothman, 1983).

This example demonstrates the need to identify the concepts that are part of the disciplines which are used in midwifery practice. This example also demonstrates the need to observe or investigate the operation of the concepts and theories from other disciplines in practice and to ask questions about the ways in which these concepts and theories are applied.

All the theorists discussed in Chapter 6 provide evidence of the theoretical base for their theory development. In all cases, to a greater or lesser extent, these theorists have all based their work on pre-existing theory in other disciplines. In their discussion of Mercer's work, Bee and Oetting (1989) refer to her use of theory from the fields of social interactionism and psychology:

> Early in Mercer's research, she drew from Mead's interactionist theory of self and Von Bertalanffy's general systems theory. As her research developed into attainment of the maternal role, she also combined the work of Werner and Erikson with Burr and associates' theory to develop a theoretical framework of role theory from an interactionist approach. (Bee and Oetting, 1989, p. 293)

Mercer (1986) describes in detail the theoretical sources for the 14 variables that she examines in her work on attainment of the maternal role (see Chapter 6). These sources range across a large number of disciplines, including psychology, sociology, anthropology, medicine and others and include reference to different schools of thought within these disciplines. Having identified these concepts in the literature of a range of disciplines, Mercer then went on to test the importance of each of these concepts, in particular that of age, in attainment of the maternal role (Mercer, 1986). Similarly, Ball (1989) describes theory on coping and support systems as the basic theoretical framework for her research on the influence of postnatal care on the adjustment to motherhood.

Deductive theory is also obtained from research in other fields. This research may identify factors or variables which may be important in understanding midwifery care. For example, Ball (1989) refers to research which has identified factors which may affect coping and stress, including anxious personality and marital tension. These variables were then incorporated by Ball (1989) into a study which sought to identify relationships between maternal adjustment, a range of variables identified from pre-existing research and theory, and midwifery care (see Chapter 6).

Theory from other disciplines may also be used to construct models or theories of midwifery practice. Littlewood (1989) provides an example of this method of theory development in relation to care of the childbearing woman. This is also the approach that was taken by theorists such as Roy and Orem in their work to develop their systems and developmental models of nursing (Pearson and Vaughan, 1986). Littlewood (1989) draws on sociological theory relating to the sick role and anthropological theory relating to culture to develop a framework, described as the Generalised Nursing Model. The use of this model is illustrated in relation to the care of a woman with pre-eclampsia, as discussed in Chapters 4 and 7. The understanding of the cultural interpretation of the signs and symptoms of pre-eclampsia made by the woman is dependent on an understanding of the meaning of these signs and symptoms within her culture:

> Social and cultural factors always play a part in the experience, aetiology, and course of the illness (Kleinmann, 1980). The illness experience is the product of the pathological process but also the understanding of health and sickness which the patient has derived from folk beliefs, past experience of sickness and her knowledge of professional medicine. (Littlewood, 1989, p. 223).

In this identification of the importance of the concept of culture to the understanding of ill-health and, in addition, to pregnancy and health Littlewood (1989) has provided a useful starting-point for the development of theories about the interaction of culture, midwifery practice and the outcomes of pregnancy. This process could result in refinement, development and testing of the model that is proposed.

Use of theory in the form of nursing models

In Chapter 7 the evidence that midwives have adapted and applied nursing models from midwifery practice was considered. This discussion showed that midwives found the concepts from which the models are constructed helpful in their own practice. For example, Methven (1986a) demonstrates the utility of Orem's model of self-care in the antenatal care of the childbearing woman. She argues that the underlying self-care philosophy of this model, which is based on respect for the individual, fits very well with midwifery practice. The type of relationship that the model describes between the nurse (or midwife) and the patient (or childbearing woman), which is one of partnership, in which the nurse acts to compensate for those activities that the individual is unable (for what ever reasons) to perform, is also one which is central to midwifery care:

> The analysis of the nurse's role, delineated by Orem, would appear to be wholly consistent with the concept of the midwife being 'with the mother' in order to 'help' her during a normal pregnancy,

delivery and puerperium. In this way the status of the mother is not reduced to that of 'patient' and the ideal of 'partnership of care' remains possible….(Methven, 1986a, p. 15)

This model also has as a central feature the promotion of health, which is a key concept in midwifery practice. Other models have been used by other midwives. In all cases, questions need to be asked about the extent to which the philosophy and theory which inform the model and the four concepts of person, health, environment and practice are applicable to midwifery.

Spires (1991), for example, argues that the Neuman Systems Model is applicable to midwifery care because it is concerned with health and the ability of the individual to cope with changes in health status, such as those that occur in pregnancy which, while it may be a state of health, involves changes in bodily function as well as in social and psychological functions. This model also places the individual firmly within their social context and requires a detailed assessment of the environment within which the person lives. Ball (1987) has demonstrated the importance of the social context of the woman's life on her adaptation to motherhood, which provides support for the value of the Neuman model to care of the childbearing woman.

Castledine and Jones (1987), on the other hand, consider that the Roy Adaptation Model is of use in the care of the childbearing woman. This view is supported by the work of Fawcett and her associates (Fawcett (1990), who have developed a research programme built on the Roy Adaptation Model. These authors argue that this model is appropriate because of its identification of the four modes of adaptation: physiology, self-concept, role function and interdependence, all of which are important during pregnancy and childbirth. The role that the model ascribes to the nurse or midwife, which is to intervene and modify the focal, contextual and residual foci (as far as is possible), is also a role which is congruent with the role of the midwife. Methven (1986a), however, argues that this model emphasises deviation from the normal and problem identification, which conflicts with the view of pregnancy being seen as a normal state as well as containing concepts from psychology and adaptation which require a significant knowledge base, and which together led her to reject use of this model.

Use of nursing models in midwifery practice has been discussed further in Chapter 7. It appears from this discussion that a number of models which have been used in midwifery practice have been found to be applicable. In passing, it is perhaps worth commenting on the vast range of nursing models. Chinn and Jacob (1991) identify 19 theories of nursing and Marriner-Tomey (1989) 26, so there are a great many that midwives appear not to have applied and tested in midwifery care (although the 26 discussed by Marriner-Tomey (1989) include Wiedenbach and Mercer). Before these models can be applied in midwifery care they need to be examined carefully in relation to their underlying philosophies and concepts. Questions then need to be asked about the extent to which the philosophy and concepts of the model are congruent with the picture or model of care of the childbearing woman held by a midwife or by a team of midwives.

Literature on or about midwifery

The third strand to the deductive identification of concepts, theories and models involves the examination of literature specifically on midwifery. Such an examination aims to identify within that literature the values and concepts held by midwives which may then be tested and related together in the process of theory-building.

Several of the theorists discussed earlier used this approach to identify the concepts that are central to midwifery. Lehrman (1981) describes the process that she adopted to identify the concepts which she then examined in a study of antenatal care:

> Some categories were developed following a review of articles from professional journals written by nurse-midwives during the past 25 years. These articles contained a consistent reoccurrence of concepts considered to be aspects of nurse-midwifery practice. These were extracted from the literature and grouped, resulting in eight aspects of nurse-midwifery practice. (Lehrman, 1981, p. 29)

The concepts that Lehrman (1981) identified, in this painstaking way, were: continuity of care; family-centred care; education and counselling as part of care; non-interventionist care; flexibility in care; participative care; consumer advocacy; and time. It might be suggested that this list provides a starting point for midwives in Britain to identify the concepts that are evident in the British literature. To what extent are these concepts the same as those found in the British literature on midwifery practice? In what ways does this list differ from the concepts that might be found to be central in the British literature on midwifery?

Lehrman (1987) provides further evidence of the utility of this approach to the identification of shared concepts in a study of care in labour based on the Nurse-Midwifery Practice Model. She describes the development of this model as being partly based on the identification of the concepts which are included in the philosophy of the American College of Nurse-Midwives. Thompson *et al.* (1989) have described the process of identifying concepts, again based initially on the above philosophy. From the philosophy these authors identified seven concepts of nurse-midwifery practice:

> ...nurse-midwifery is safe
> is satisfying
> respects human dignity
> respects cultural and ethnic diversity
> promotes self-determination
> is family centred
> promotes health

(Thompson *et al.*, 1989, p. 122)

This list immediately identifies the differences between the concepts identified in the philosophy and those identified by Lehrman (1981) in the literature. This difference may reflect changes in thinking between 1981 and 1989 or it may reflect differences between those who draft philosophies and the broader cross-section of nurse-midwives who may write articles.

Thompson *et al.* (1989) go on to describe the process they went through to refine, define and develop indicators for these concepts. This involved making video-tapes of antenatal visits, which were then reviewed by a panel of nurse-midwives and a researcher, who was not a nurse-midwife, who identified indicators of each of the concepts. A number of nurse-midwives then completed a questionnaire about what they thought was special about nurse-midwifery care. The indicators identified by the panel were combined with the results from the questionnaires and the results of a literature search regarding client views of nurse-midwifery practice. The concepts and indicators were then reviewed by several different groups of nurse-midwives and finally, 'the group indicated that the concepts were sufficiently comprehensive to delineate the nurse-midwifery care process, that the definitions were essentially accurate, and that the concept components were adequate' (Thompson *et al.*, 1989, p. 122). During this process it was decided that the concepts of 'respects human dignity' and 'promotes self-determination' were so similar that they were merged and formed one concept: respecting human dignity and self-determination. The delineation of these concepts and identification of the indicators of these concepts (see Chapter 2) in practice can now be used to assess whether these five concepts do in fact describe nurse-midwifery practice or not.

Written material on midwifery indicates both the underlying theory and knowledge that is used in midwifery but it also demonstrates the values, beliefs and attitudes that midwives hold about society, midwifery and care of the childbearing woman. In Chapter 5, material, including information from textbooks, other books and philosophies of care, was presented which demonstrates the values held by midwives. This small review indicated the range of concepts that are held by midwives and which midwives consider inform their practice. Although, as Thompson *et al.* (1989) demonstrate, this approach to concept identification and validation may be time-consuming, it has the potential to provide a means of identifying the values and concepts that midwives hold in common.

INDUCTIVE APPROACHES

The identification of concepts, theories and models using an inductive approach starts from the practice of midwifery rather than the disciplines or literature which are used in that care. Three inductive approaches may be identified: those associated with qualitative research; those which involve efforts to expose shared meanings; and those which focus on the exposure of practice theory.

Qualitative research

The main aim of qualitative research is to describe the world from the perspective of the participants in that world. The person who is collecting information, or undertaking research and collecting data, therefore uses methods which enable the individuals, who are being observed in various ways, to demonstrate or report their feelings, attitudes, beliefs and views about their world (Field and Morse, 1985). This approach contrasts with the deductive method in which the researcher determines from the literature and available theory the concepts that are important in relation to that aspect of care. In deductive research a questionnaire or some other measurement tool would then be developed which would be used to measure the existence of the concepts in practice. Lehrman (1981) provides one example of this approach to testing concepts. In Lehrman's (1981) case, she tape-recorded antenatal visits, which were then quantitatively analysed using the concepts she had identified in the literature.

In contrast, in inductive research, data are collected about an area of interest by unstructured observation, open or semi-structured interviews and by other means. The aim is to provide the subjects with the opportunity to express their own views rather than being limited, for example by a questionnaire, to the issues that the researcher has decided are important. Through this means the informants have the opportunity to identify issues and aspects of their lives or their midwifery care. The researcher using a deductive approach might never have identified these aspects if they did not form part of the deductive theory on which their study was built. Qualitative research therefore has the potential to uncover people's real feelings about their lives, their midwifery care or, for midwives, to describe the reality of being a midwife.

Through the systematic collection and analysis of data, categories are identified which are further refined and identified as concepts which form part of the world-view of that group of people. Once these concepts have been described, it is then possible to go on to test their validity and meaning for other groups of people through deductive research (research which is developed, or deduced, from the concepts identified in the qualitative research). This description indicates that qualitative research can be described, using Dickoff and James's (1992) classification (see Chapter 2), as factor-isolating theory, as it is aimed at uncovering the factors or concepts that make up individuals' theories and models of their world.

In midwifery there is a large number of studies which have used this approach to concept identification. Kirkham (1989) undertook a study of the flow of information between midwives and women during labour in which she observed 113 labours and collected information by taking notes: 'I wanted to know what actually happens in labour and therefore chose observation as my principal research method. I undertook continuous observations of labour during which I took written notes' (Kirkham, 1989, p. 117). In addition, Kirkham (1989) undertook a large number of interviews with the women who were pregnant, the women whose labours had been observed and midwives. Analysis involved categorisation of the observations. As this study started from a question about information in labour the categories developed reflect this. The categories identified include: social class, labelling of patients, and the order of the ward; the inhibiting effect of senior staff (on information-giving) and verbal asepsis. This last concept Kirkham (1989) describes as a means that the midwives used so that they did not have to engage with the worries or concerns expressed by the women. For example:

Woman: Is there only one sort of injection?
Sister: Don't be thinking six hours ahead or four hours ahead. See how it goes. I say see how it goes. Changes subject. (Kirkham, 1989, p. 125)

The identification of the concept of verbal asepsis by Kirkham (1989) could probably not have occurred from a consideration of pre-existing theory (although reference to the work of Menzies (1960) discussed in Chapter 2 might have led to the proposition that such a concept could exist). Examination of the literature on midwifery (for example, that reviewed above by Lehrman (1981) and Thompson *et al.* (1989)) would suggest that this is a concept which is very foreign to midwives, who emphasise participation and sharing of information in the rhetoric about midwifery care. The identification of this concept opens up the possibility, now that further data may be collected about care in labour, to discover if this concept is found in settings other than those investigated by Kirkham (1989). This data may be collected in formal research studies but it may also be collected by all midwives who are involved in care of women during childbirth. For example, what language is used in the labour ward where you are working, and does this language encourage the woman to be a partner in her care? This study illustrates the value of qualitative studies to identify concepts. These concepts and the factors which support or reduce the impact of the concept should then be explored through further research which would provide tested practice-derived theory.

In another qualitative study, which investigated the lived experience of postnatal depression, Beck (1993) acted as a facilitator in a postnatal support group and interviewed women attending the group, about their experiences of postnatal depression. Beck (1993) provides a detailed description of the process which she used to analyse the interviews and develop theoretical constructs (concepts) from the data. A theory of postnatal depression is proposed from the data which describes women as moving through four stages in their experience of postnatal depression, an experience of teetering on the edge between sanity and insanity. These stages or concepts are: encountering terror; dying of self; struggling to survive and regaining control. Again, as with Kirkham's (1989) study, these concepts describe the process of postnatal depression from the viewpoint of the women involved.

Oakley (1979; 1980), in an extensive study of first-time mothers, describes both the research process, the process of theory construction and the data which are collected in qualitative research. In *Becoming a Mother* Oakley (1979) uses excerpts from the interviews that she and another researcher held with women during pregnancy and following the birth. These interviews were partly structured but the unstructured sections demonstrate in great detail the attitudes, expectations and experiences of these women during this process of becoming a mother.

Other qualitative studies have been referred to in earlier chapters which used open or semi-structured tape-recorded interviews. Weitz and Sullivan (1985) gathered information about the models of care held by lay midwives, through interviews with the midwives, and Benoit (1989) used the same method in her study of the work of midwives in different settings in Newfoundland and Labrador. McCrea (1993) has used this method, interviewing midwives, to explore poor relationships between midwives and mothers, while Bowler (1993) examined one aspect of communication, stereotyping, in her study using this method. McCrea (1993) identifies the concept of the midwives' self-confidence in their role as a key issue in their relationships with women. Their self-confidence was affected by their ability to develop relationships with women and their partners. Bowler (1993) adds to the understanding of this process in her analysis of the ways in which midwives stereotype women from another culture. Again, in all these examples, the demonstration of these concepts enables the further testing of the concepts in practice and through research.

Identifying shared meanings

Implicit in much of the discussion in this book has been the need for all midwives to make explicit to themselves, and others, the concepts which form their pictures of midwifery care. It has been suggested that this process will then enable discussion about concepts which are shared and those that are not held in common. Most midwifery care is provided within the context of organisations, hospitals or teams. There are very few midwives in Britain who work in isolated practice (although like many primary health care practitioners many community midwives may not be working in teams which have much face-to-face interaction). Midwifery practice involves teamwork to a greater or lesser extent and teamwork will be facilitated for those teams or other work groups if they understand each others' approaches to care and come to some understanding of their shared or different approaches.

A number of authors provide evidence of ways in which shared meanings may be identified and developed. Henderson (1990) describes a process which occurred over a period of four years in a maternity unit. This process began with the introduction of birth plans and individualised care. This was followed by discussion of the philosophy of care, 'with discussions of the beliefs and values of mothers and midwives being important considerations' (Henderson, 1990, p. 64). Following an examination and rejection of current models it was

decided that the midwives would develop their own model based on
their own care practices. Working groups were set up in which staff
identified the 'elements of care' (Henderson, 1990, p. 66) and decided
that they wanted to base the model on Maslow's hierarchy of needs.
Using other literature (discussed in Chapter 7) the Human Needs Model
of Midwifery was devised and used in practice. At the same time, 'the
midwives highlighted the need to review existing documentation'
(Henderson, 1990, p. 65) and developed new documentation which,
presumably, facilitated the use of the model. Methven (1989) has
demonstrated the constraints imposed by inappropriate records on the
model used. There is a need for clear, accurate, up-to-date records
which support the utilisation of the shared model in practice.
Henderson concludes that the model 'affords midwives the opportunity
to discuss their values and beliefs, thus allowing them to control the
care they give. The model presented here reflects the views, philosophies and assumptions of one group of midwives. It is a framework
serving to guide practice, a structured way to plan, implement and
evaluate care' (Henderson, 1990, pp. 66–7).

This description of the process of developing shared meanings, from
the meanings of individual midwives, which took four years, illustrates
the time that is needed to work through this process of change. Mayes
(1987) and Smith (1991) provide two further descriptions of the
process of uncovering meanings which provide additional information
about the meaning ascribed by the midwives to the different concepts
(see Chapter 7).

From the field of care of the elderly, Wright (1986; 1990) provides
much sound advice about the process of uncovering the models of care
held by nurses which is equally applicable to midwifery. Wright (1990)
describes the process involved in developing a model to guide practice
in a unit described as being an ordinary one, staffed by people who had
had few educational opportunities. Many meetings were held, which
were facilitated by staff who had joint appointments in the unit and in
education, and the philosophy of the team was identified through discussion and reading of relevant articles and books. The model was then
used to guide practice, the education of staff and students and research
activity in the unit. Wright (1986) comments that models for practice
must be relevant to the staff on a unit and the type of people they are
caring for:

1 Models must be built, described and used in language that is
   accessible to all levels of nursing staff.

2 A nursing model which focuses solely on the patient, and neglects
   or underestimates the nurses themselves and the social backcloth
   of the hospital and community, is of little value. (Wright, 1986,
   p. 40)

Smith (1991) illustrates the importance of these issues in the development of the Newborne model which considers the woman and
fetus/infant in the context of her extended family and the wider society
and cultural values. A care plan completed by the woman is described
as being worded in a user-friendly way to encourage participation and
to prevent the language being a barrier between midwives and childbearing women.

Wright (1986) comments that models should be constantly developing and changing and that change is, in a way, built into the process of
model development. The thinking about practice which development
of a model entails leads to questions being asked about many areas of
practice. This questioning may lead to research and modification or development of the model. The approach to model development that
Wright (1990) describes, which is rooted in the practice setting and is
largely unpredictable, is essentially concerned with challenging practice and discovering the reasons for different aspects of practice. This
approach is a form of change management which starts from the staff
on a unit rather than from a pre-existing theory or model, and is an
example of the use of an inductive approach to theory development
involving a large number of practitioners working in one setting.

Practice theory

Qualitative research methods and the process of identifying shared
meanings can both be described as approaches to theory development
which are within the naturalism paradigm (Vaughan, 1992). The
process of exploring practice through description and identification of
the elements in that practice may be described as occurring within the
paradigm of critical social theory, or it may simply be considered as the
best starting-place for identifying the concepts that midwives demonstrate in their practice.

The important point here is the demonstration or description of the
concepts in practice. Rather than midwives describing what they think
they should do, the emphasis here is on the midwives describing or
demonstrating what they actually do in practice. These descriptions aim
to identify the midwives' theories-in-use rather than their espoused

theories-in-action (Agyris and Schön, 1974). Such espoused theories are formed of the past learning of the individual and are the sort of theories that people will describe if asked how they would behave in certain circumstances. It might be argued that it is espoused theories that are found in philosophies and in other writings. What is more important, however, is the way that midwives and others act in practice which, Agyris and Schön (1974), argue, demonstrates their theories-in-use. As discussed in Chapter 3 there may be organisational reasons (in addition to educational or other reasons) for any disparity between espoused theories and theories-in-use. For example, midwives in the project described earlier held the theory (espoused theory) that individualised care of the childbearing woman was very important. In practice their care was constrained by organisational policies and other demands so that there was a gap between this espoused theory and the theory-in-use that the midwives demonstrated in their practice (Bryar, 1985). This type of observation is, of course, an argument for change at all points in the action framework, if real change is to be achieved.

Agyris and Schön (1974) describe a process which helps individuals to identify their theories-in-use (or practice theories). Individuals are asked to write about 'a challenging intervention or interaction with one or more individuals that (1) you have already experienced or (2) you might expect to experience in the near future' (Agyris and Schön, 1974, p. 41). The description identifies on one half of the paper what was going on in the writer's mind during the incident, and the other half describes, as closely as possible, the content of the intervention. The description of the incident is then discussed in a group setting. Reflection by the individual and discussion with the group helps in the identification of the underlying attitudes and concepts held by the writer. Awareness of these attitudes, concepts and the behaviours or actions, which are associated with these concepts, can then lead to change, modification or conscious testing of the concepts and theories in practice. Agyris and Schön (1974) are concerned with achieving change rather than undertaking this activity as an aid to theory-building but many midwives, seeking to provide a new form of midwifery care, would probably agree with these authors' aim for this process:

Understanding how we diagnose and construct our experience, take action, and monitor our behaviour while simultaneously achieving our goals is crucial to understanding and enhancing effectiveness. If we learn to behave differently and to make these new behaviours stick, we will begin to create a new world. (Agyris and Schön, 1974, p. xi)

The importance of the everyday practice base as the starting-point for theory development has been demonstrated in the work of Benner (1984). Benner starts from descriptions of practice to identify what it means to be a nurse and the competences involved in that practice (Benner, 1984; Benner and Wrubel, 1989). Through the collection and examination of descriptions of practice Benner seeks to identify the elements which combine together in practice at the different levels of competence. It can be seen that, while this approach rests on the examination in detail of practice descriptions, it is also an approach which is formed, and depends on, deductive theory for the broad framework of analysis.

The process described by Agyris and Schön (1974) may be described as a process of story-telling. Story-telling is an approach that has been used by Fairbairn and Mead (1993a and 1993b) in exploring ethical dilemmas or the operation of ethical concepts in nursing. These authors describe in detail the process they use to explore these dilemmas. Group participants are given stories of practice incidents which present moral dilemmas and are asked to think themselves into the story. Having thought themselves into the story they are then asked to write, as openly as possible, about the story. A discussion then takes place at which the participants draw out from their own stories and the original story the ethical issues in the story: that is, they identify the ethical concepts and the actions that resulted from these concepts. In a similar way, midwives could write stories about their practice and then use those stories to identify the midwifery concepts in that practice.

Fairbairn and Mead (1993b) comment on the grieving that this process of sharing stories can entail as memories of similar ethical dilemmas suffered by participants are reawakened. This would have to be remembered in the use of story-telling in midwifery, even though the stories would not necessarily be about distressing incidents. It is as important to identify the concepts that are demonstrated in the supportive talk between midwife and woman during an antenatal visit as it is to identify the concepts in more distressing situations. Exposure of concepts of practice involves thinking and reflection which may be unfamiliar to some and even avoided. It is a process that requires support which may be provided by a group, which 'must be a group that helps its members to learn' (Agyris and Schön, 1974), or by individual forms of support such as mentorship (Morton-Cooper and Palmer, 1993).

Exposure of practice theory through description and teasing-out of the concepts implicit in the actions described appears to have the potential to assist midwives in speaking about midwifery practice. Sharing of these descriptions may help to identify shared concepts as well as differences in thinking. These concepts can then be further explored through further story-telling, observation of practice and research.

Summary

 In this chapter, the aim has been to draw together the discussion and descriptions in earlier chapters in a consideration of a number of approaches to concept identification and theory building in and for midwifery practice. Two main approaches have been described: deductive approaches and inductive approaches. Deductive approaches include: use of theory from other disciplines; the use of theory in the form of nursing models; and the use of literature on and about midwifery. Inductive approaches include: qualitative research; identification of shared meanings; and practice theory. Different approaches will be suitable for different situations and for different people. Deductive and inductive approaches and combination of these approaches provide enormous possibilities for the further development of theory of and for midwifery practice. This future development will help further to answer the question with which this book commenced: How do I care? How do you care?

REFERENCES

Aaronson, L. S. 1987. Nurse-Midwives and Obstetricians: Alternative models of care and client 'fit'. *Research in Nursing and Health* 10: 217–26.

Abel, S. and Kearns, R. A. 1991. Birth Places: A geographical perspective on planned home birth in New Zealand. *Social Science and Medicine* 33(7): 825–34.

Ackerman, B. 1986. Midwives – past, present and future. In Claxton, R. (ed), *Birth Matters. Issues and alternatives in childbirth*. Ch. 4: pp. 62–74. Unwin Paperbacks, London.

Adair, J. 1986. *Effective Teambuilding*. Pan Books, London.

Adams, M., Armstrong-Esther, C., Bryar, R., Duberley, J., Strong, G. and Ward, E. 1981. The Nursing Process in Midwifery: Trial run. *Nursing Mirror* 151 (9): 26–7.

Aggleton, P. and Chalmers, H. 1986. *Nursing Models and the Nursing Process*. Macmillan, London.

Aggleton, P. and Chalmers, H. 1987. Models of Nursing, Nursing Practice and Nurse Education. *Journal of Advanced Nursing* 12(5): 573–81.

Agyris, C. and Schön, D. A. 1974. *Theory in Practice. Increasing Professional Effectiveness*. Jossey-Bass Publishers, San Francisco.

Alexander, J. E. 1989. From Novice to Expert: Excellence and power in clinical nursing practice. In Marriner-Tomey, A. (ed.), *Nursing Theorists and Their Work*. 2nd Edition. Ch. 16: pp. 187–99. The C. V. Mosby Co., St Louis.

Ament, L. A. 1989. Maternal Tasks of the Puerperium Reidentified. *JOGNN, Journal of Obstetric, Gynecologic and Neonatal Nursing* 19(4): 330–5.

Andreano, R. 1993. Reflections on the Economist and Health Economics in an International Setting. *Social Science and Medicine* 36(2): 137–41.

Arms, S. 1981. *Immaculate Deception*. Bantam Books, New York.

Arney, W. R. 1982. *Power and the Profession of Obstetrics*. The University of Chicago Press, Chicago.

Association for Improvements in the Maternity Services, 1992. Childbirth Care – Users' Views. Submission to the House of Commons Health Committee 1991. AIMS, Iver, Buckinghamshire.

Association of Radical Midwives. 1986. *The Vision: Proposals for the future of the maternity services*. The Association of Radical Midwives, Ormskirk, Lancashire.

Auvenshine, M. A. and Enriquez, M. G. 1990. *Comprehensive Maternity Nursing*. 2nd Edition. Jones and Bartlett Publishers, Boston.

Ball, J. A. 1981. The Effects of the Present Patterns of Maternity Care upon the Emotional Needs of Mothers: I, II and III. *Midwives Chronicle* 95(1120): 150–4; (1121): 198–202; (1122): 231–3.

Ball, J. A. 1987. *Reactions to Motherhood. The role of postnatal care*. Cambridge University Press, Cambridge.

Ball, J. A. 1989. Postnatal Care and Adjustment to Motherhood. In Robinson, S. and Thomson, A. (eds), *Midwives, Research and Childbirth*. Volume I. Ch. 8: 154–75. Chapman and Hall, London.

Ball, J. A., Flint, C., Garvey, M., Jackson-Baker, A., Page, L. and Bryans, B. 1992. *Who's Left Holding the Baby? An organisational framework for making the most of midwifery services*. The Nuffield Institute for Health Services Studies, University of Leeds, Leeds.

Ball, J. A. and Hughes, D. 1993. Quality Assurance in Maternity care. In Bennett, V. R. and Brown, L. K. (eds), 1993. *Myles Textbook for Midwives*. 12th Edition. Ch. 52: pp. 793–808. Churchill Livingstone, Edinburgh.

Barclay, L., Andre, C. A. and Glover, P. A. 1989. Women's Business: The challenge of childbirth. *Midwifery* 5(3): 122–33.

Beck, C. T. 1993. Teetering on the Edge: A substantive theory of postpartum depression. *Nursing Research* 42(1): 42–8.

Bee, A. M. and Oetting, S. 1989. Ramona T Mercer: Maternal role attainment. In Marriner-Tomey, A. (ed), *Nursing Theorists and Their Work*. 2nd Edition. Ch. 24: pp. 292–306. The C. V. Mosby Co., St Louis.

Belbin, R. M. 1981. *Management Teams: Why they succeed or fail*. Heinemann, London.

Benner, P. 1984. *From Novice to Expert. Excellence and power in clinical nursing practice*. Addison-Wesley Publishing Co, Menlo Park, California.

Benner, P. and Wrubel, J. 1989. *The Primacy of Caring. Stress and coping in health and illness*. Addison-Wesley Publishing Co., Menlo Park, California.

Bennett, V. R. and Brown, L. K. (eds), 1993. *Myles Textbook for Midwives*. 12th Edition. Churchill Livingstone, Edinburgh.

Benoit, C. M. 1987. Midwives in Passage: A case study of occupational change. PhD thesis. Unpublished. University of Toronto, Toronto.

Benoit, C. 1989. The Professional Socialisation of Midwives: Balancing art and science. *Sociology of Health and Illness* 11(2): 160–80.

Benoit, C. 1992. Midwives in Comparative Perspective: Professionalism in small organizations. *Current Research on Occupations and Professions* 7: 203–20.

Berger, P. and Luckmann, T. 1967. *The Social Construction of Reality*. Penguin Books, Harmondsworth, Middlesex.

Boud, D., Keogh, R. and Walker, D. 1985. *Reflection: Turning experience into learning*. Kogan Page, London.

Bowler, I. 1993. 'They're Not the Same as Us': Midwives' stereotypes of South Asian descent maternity patients. *Sociology of Health and Illness* 15(2): 157–78.

Brackbill, Y., Rice, J. and Young, D. 1984. *Birth Trap. The legal low-down on high-tech obstetrics*. The C. V. Mosby Company, St Louis.

Bradshaw, J. and Whitfield, S. 1986. *Planned Individualised Care of Mother, Baby and Family Unit*. ENB Learning Resources Unit, Sheffield.

Brearley, S. 1990. *Patient Participation: The literature*. Scutari Press, Harrow.

Breen, D. 1975. *The Birth of a First Child: Towards an understanding of femininity*. Tavistock Publications, London.

Bryar, R. and Strong, G. 1983. Trial run – continued. *Nursing Mirror* 157(15): 45–8.

Bryar, R. 1985. A Study of the Introduction of the Nursing Process in a Maternity Unit. MPhil thesis. Unpublished. Southbank Polytechnic, London.

Bryar, R. 1987. The Nursing Process: A literature review. *Midwifery* 3(3): 109–16.

Bryar, R. 1988. Midwifery and Models of Care. *Midwifery* 4(3): 111–17.

Bryar, R. 1991a. Research and Individualised Care in Midwifery. In Robinson, S. and Thomson, A. M. (eds), *Midwives, Research and Childbirth*. Volume 2. Ch. 3: pp. 48–71. Chapman and Hall, London.

Bryar, R. 1991b. 'Since the Centre Started I am a Different Woman': Report of a WHO Fellowship visit to the Netherlands. Teamcare Valleys, Welsh Office, Cardiff.

Buckenham, J. E. and McGrath, G. 1983. *The Social Reality of Nursing*. ADIS Health Service Press, Sydney.

Carper, B. A. 1992. Fundamental Patterns of Knowing in Nursing. In Nicholl, L. H. (ed), *Perspectives on Nursing Theory*. 2nd Edition. Ch. 19: pp. 216–24. J. B. Lippincott Co., Philadelphia.

Carter, D. 1992. A Philosophy of Care. Unpublished. Mid Trent College of Nursing and Midwifery, Faculty of Midwifery.

Carty, E. M. and Tier, D. T. 1989. Birth Planning. A reality-based script for building confidence. *Journal of Nurse-Midwifery* 34(3): 111–14.

Carveth, J. A. 1987. Conceptual Models in Nurse-Midwifery. *Journal of Nurse-Midwifery* 32(1): 20–5.

Castledine, G. and Jones, K. 1987. Model Pregnancies. *Senior Nurse* 7(1): 7–8.

Chalmers, I., Oakley, A. and MacFarlane, A. 1980. Perinatal Health Services: An immodest proposal. *British Medical Journal* 280 (6,217): 842–5.

Chapman, C. M. 1985. *Theory of Nursing: Practical application*. Harper and Row, London.

Chin, R. and Benne, K. D. 1976. General Strategies for Effecting Changes in Human Systems. In Bennis, W. G., Benne, K. D., Chin, R. and Corey, K. E. *The Planning of Change*. 3rd Edition. Holt, Rinehart and Winston, New York. Cited by Hegyvary, S. T. 1982. *The Change to Primary Nursing: A cross-cultural view of nursing practice*. The C. V. Mosby Company, St Louis.

Chinn, P. L. and Kramer, M. K. 1991. Theory and Nursing: A systematic approach. Mosby Year Book, St Louis.

Clark, M. 1986. Action and Reflection: Practice and theory in nursing. *Journal of Advanced Nursing* 11(1): 3–11.

Comaroff, J. 1977. Conflicting Paradigms of Pregnancy: Managing ambiguity in ante-natal encounters. In Davis, A. and Horobin, G. (eds), *Medical Encounters: The Experience of Illness and Treatment*. Ch. 8: pp. 115–34. Croom Helm, London.

Combes, G. and Schonveld, A. 1992. *Life will Never be the Same Again. Learning to be a first time parent*. Health Education Authority, London.

Cornford, F. M. 1946. Plato's *Theory of Knowledge*. Kegan Paul, Trench, Trubner and Co, London.

Cranley, M. S. 1981. Development of a Tool for the Measurement of Maternal Attachment during Pregnancy. *Nursing Research* 30(5): 281–84.

Cronenwett, L. and Brickman, P. 1983. Models of Helping and Coping in Childbirth. *Nursing Research* 32(2): 84–8.

Currell, R. 1990. The Organisation of Midwifery Care. In Alexander, J., Levy, V. and Roch, S. (eds), *Midwifery Care. Antenatal care. A research-based approach*. Ch. 2: pp. 20–41. Macmillan, London.

Danko, M., Hunt, N. E., Marich, J. E., Marriner-Tomey, A., McCreary, C. A. and Stuart, M. 1989. Ernestine Wiedenbach: The helping art of clinical nursing. In Marriner-Tomey, A. (ed.), *Nursing Theorists and their Work*. 2nd Edition. Ch. 20: pp. 240–52. The C. V. Mosby Co., St Louis.

Davies, C. and Francis, A. 1976. Perceptions of Structure in National Health Service Hospitals. In Stacy, M. (ed.), *The Sociology of the NHS*: 120-39. Sociological Review Monograph 22. University of Keele, Keele.

Davies, C. 1979. Organization Theory and the Organization of Health Care: A comment on the literature. *Social Science and Medicine* 13A(4): 413–22.

Davies, J. and Evans, F. 1991. Newcastle Community Midwifery Care Project. In Robinson, S. and Thomson, A. M. (eds), *Midwives, Research and Childbirth*. Volume II. Ch. 5: pp. 104–39. Chapman and Hall, London.

Davis, E. 1987. *Heart and Hands. A midwife's guide to pregnancy and birth*. 2nd Edition. Celestial Arts, Berkeley, California.

DeMeester, D., Lauer, T., Neal, S. E. and Williams, S. 1989. Virginia Henderson. Definition of Nursing. In Marriner-Tomey, A. (ed.), *Nursing Theorists and Their Work*. 2nd Edition. Ch. 8: pp. 80–92. The C. V. Mosby Co., St Louis.

Department of Health. 1991. *The Health of the Nation. A consultative document for health in England*. HMSO, London.

Department of Health. 1993a. *Changing Childbirth*. Part I: Report of the Expert Maternity Group. HMSO, London.

Department of Health. 1993b. *Changing Childbirth* Part II: Survey of Good Communications Practice in Maternity Services. HMSO, London.

DeVries, R. G. 1993. A Cross-national View of the Status of Midwives. In Riska, E. and Wegar, K. (eds) *Gender, Work and Medicine: Women and the medical division of labour*. SAGE Publications, London.

Dickoff, J. and James, P. 1992. A Theory of Theories: A position paper. In Nicholl, L. H. (ed.), *Perspectives on Nursing Theory*. 2nd Edition. Ch. 8: pp. 99–111. J. B. Lippincott Co., Philadelphia.

Dickoff, J., James, P. and Wiedenbach, E. 1992a. Theory in a Practice Discipline, Part I: Practice orientated theory. In Nicholl, L. H. (ed.), *Perspectives on Nursing Theory*. 2nd Edition. Ch. 46: pp. 468–500. J. B. Lippincott Co., Philadelphia.

Dickoff, J., James, P. and Wiedenbach, E. 1992b. Theory in a Practice Discipline, Part II: Practice oriented research. In Nicholl, L. H. (ed.), *Perspectives on Nursing Theory*. 2nd Edition. Ch. 53: pp. 585–98. J. B. Lippincott Co., Philadelphia.

Dick-Read, G. 1987. *Childbirth without Fear: The original approach to natural childbirth*. 5th Edition. Harper and Row, New York.

Dines, A. and Cribb, A. (eds), 1993. *Health Promotion. Concepts and practice*. Blackwell Scientific Publications, Oxford.

Distance Learning Centre. 1992. *Midwifery Update Modules 1–9*. Distance Learning Centre, South Bank University, London.

Donnison, J. 1988. Midwives and Medical Men. 2nd Edition. Historical Publications, London.

Downe, S. 1991. 'The Midwife as Practitioner': Midwifery Standards – Uniformity or Quality? *Midwives Chronicle and Nursing Notes* 104(1,236): 3–4.

Dubos, R. 1960. *Mirage of Health*. George Allen and Unwin, London. Cited by McKeown, T. 1979. *The Role of Medicine: Dream, mirage or nemesis?* Basil Blackwell, Oxford.

Dunkerley, D. 1972. *The Study of Organizations*. Routledge and Kegan Paul, London.

Dunn, S. I. and Trépanier, M.–J. 1989. Application of the Neuman Systems Model to Perinatal Nursing. In Neuman B., *The Neuman Systems Model*. 2nd Edition. Ch. 24: pp. 407–21. Appleton and Lange, Norwalk, Connecticut.

Dunnington, R. M. and Glazer, G. 1991. Maternal Identity and Early Mothering Behaviour in Previously Infertile and Never Infertile Women. *JOGNN, Journal of Obstetric, Gynecologic and Neonatal Nursing* 20(4): 309–18.

Eben, J. D., Gashti, N. N., Nation, M. J., Marriner-Tomey, A. and Nordmeyer, S. B. 1989. Dorethea E Orem. Self-Care Deficit Theory of Nursing. In Marriner-Tomey, A. (ed.), *Nursing Theorists and Their Work*. 2nd Edition. Ch. 11: pp. 118–32. The C. V. Mosby Co., St Louis.

Ehrenreich, B. and English, D. 1973. *Witches, Midwives and Nurses: A history of women healers*. Writers and Readers Publishing Cooperative, London.

Enkin, M., Keirse, M. J. N. C. and Chalmers, I. 1991. *A Guide to Effective Care in Pregnancy and Childbirth*. Oxford University Press, Oxford.

Ewles, L. and Simnett, I. 1992. *Promoting Health: A practical guide*. 2nd Edition. Scutari Press, London.

Eyer, D. E. 1993. *Mother–Infant Bonding: A scientific fiction*. Yale University Press, New Haven.

Fairbairn, G. and Mead, D. 1993a. How Nurses can Use a Story-telling Approach. *Nursing Standard* 7(32): 32–6.

Fairbairn, G. and Mead, D. 1993b. Working with the Stories Nurses Tell. *Nursing Standard* 7(31): 37–40.

Fauvel, J., Flood, R., Shortland, M. and Wilson, R. 1989. *Let Newton Be!* Oxford University Press, Oxford.

Fawcett, J. 1984. *Analysis and Evaluation of Conceptual Models of Nursing.* F. A. Davis Company, Philadelphia.

Fawcett, J. and Tulman, L. 1990. Building a Programme of research from the Roy Adaptation Model of Nursing. *Journal of Advanced Nursing* 15(6): 720–5.

Fawcett, J. 1990. Preparation for Caesarean Childbirth: Derivation of a nursing intervention from the Roy Adaptation Model. *Journal of Advanced Nursing* 15(12): 1418–25.

Fawcett, J. 1992. A Framework for Analysis and Evaluation of Conceptual Models of Nursing. In Nicholl, L. H. (ed.), *Perspectives on Nursing Theory.* 2nd Edition. Ch. 41: pp. 424–41. J. B. Lippincott Company, Philadelphia.

Fawcett, J., Pollio, N., Tully, A., Baron, M., Henklein, J. C. and Jones, R. C. 1993. Effects of Information on Adaptation to Cesarean Birth. *Nursing Research* 42(1): 49–53.

Fender, H. 1981. Midwifery Care Plan. *The Association of Radical Midwives Newsletter.* No. 11. Sept.: 10–11.

Field, P. A. 1983. An Ethnography: Four public health nurses' perspectives of nursing. *Journal of Advanced Nursing* 8(1): 3–12.

Field, P. A. and Morse, J. M. 1985. *Nursing Research: The application of qualitative approaches.* Croom Helm, London.

Field, P. A. 1990. Effectiveness and Efficacy of Antenatal Care. *Midwifery* 6(4): 215–23.

Fitzpatrick, J. J. and Whall, A. L. 1989. *Conceptual Models of Nursing: Analysis and application.* 2nd Edition. Appleton and Lange, Norwalk, Connecticut.

Flint, C. 1989. *Sensitive Midwifery.* Heinemann Nursing, Oxford.

Flint, C. 1993. *Midwifery Teams and Caseloads.* Butterworth/Heinemann Ltd, Oxford.

Freidson, E. 1970. *Professional Dominance: The social structure of medical care.* Atherton, New York.

Freidson, E. 1975. *Profession of Medicine: A study of the sociology of applied knowledge.* Dodd, Mead and Company, New York.

Garcia, J., Kilpatrick, R. and Richards, M. (eds). 1990. *The Politics of Maternity Care. Services for childbearing women in twentieth-century Britain.* Clarendon Press, London.

Garcia, J., Garforth, S. and Ayers, S. 1987. The Policy and Practice in Midwifery Study: Introduction and methods. *Midwifery* 3(1): 2–9.

Garforth, S. and Garcia, J. 1987. Admitting – A Weakness or a Strength? Routine admission of a woman in labour. *Midwifery* 3(1): 10–24.

Gaskin, I. M. 1977. *Spiritual Midwifery.* The Book Publishing Company, Summertown.

Glaser, B. G. and Strauss, A. L. 1967. *The Discovery of Grounded Theory: Strategies for qualitative research.* Aldine Publishing Co, New York.

Gonot, P. J. 1989. Imogene M. King's Conceptual Framework for Nursing. In Fitzpatrick, J. J. and Whall, A. L. (eds), *Conceptual Models of Nursing. Analysis and application.* 2nd Edition. Ch. 18: pp. 271–83. Appleton and Lange, Norwalk, Connecticut.

Goss, M. E. W. 1963. Patterns of Bureaucracy among Hospital Staff Physicians. In Freidson, E. (ed.), *The Hospital in Modern Society*. Ch. 6: pp. 170–94. Macmillan, New York.

Hakim, C. 1987. *Research Design. Strategies and choices in the design of social research*. Unwin Hyman, London.

Hall, M., MacIntyre, S. and Porter, M. 1985. *Antenatal Care Assessed. A case study of an innovation in Aberdeen*. Aberdeen University Press, Aberdeen.

Handy, C. B. 1976. *Understanding Organisations*. Penguin Books, Harmondsworth.

Hayward, J. 1975. *Information – A prescription against pain*. Royal College of Nursing, London.

Hayward, J. 1986. Report of the Nursing Process Evaluation Working Group. NERU Report No 5. Nursing Education Research Unit, Department of Nursing Studies, King's College, London.

Hegyvary, S. T. 1982. *The Change to Primary Nursing: A Cross-Cultural View of Nursing Practice*. The C. V. Mosby Company, St Louis.

Henderson, C. 1990. Models and Midwifery. In Kershaw, B. and Salvage, J. (eds), *Models for Nursing* 2. Ch. 7: pp. 57–67. Scutari Press, London.

Henderson, V. 1969. *Basic Principles of Nursing Care*. International Council of Nurses, Geneva.

Hillan, E. M. 1992. Issues in the Delivery of Midwifery Care. *Journal of Advanced Nursing* 17(3): 274–8.

HMSO. 1992. *The Patients' Charter: A charter for health*. HMSO, London.

House of Commons Health Committee. 1992. *Maternity Services,* Volume I. (Chairman Mr N. Winterton.) HMSO, London.

Hughes, D. 1988. *Midwifery and Models: A High Road to Nowhere? An evaluation of the place of theory in midwifery practice*. MIDIRS Information Pack. Number 8. August: 1–4 [un-numbered, my numbering]

Hughes, D. J. F. and Goldstone, L. A. 1989. Frameworks for Midwifery Care in Great Britain: An exploration of quality assurance. *Midwifery* 5(4): 163–71.

Hugman, R. 1991. *Power in Caring Professions*. Macmillan, London.

Hunt, S. and Symonds, A. (in press) *The Social Meaning of Midwifery*. Macmillan, London.

Inch, S. 1989. *Approaching Birth. Meeting the challenge of labour*. Green Print, London.

Independent Midwives Association. 1993. Register of Independent Midwives. Independent Midwives Association, Southampton.

International Confederation of Midwives. 1993. Position/policy statements adopted by ICN council at meeting in Vancouver – May 1993. *Midwifery* 9(3): 169–72.

Jensen, M. D., Benson, R. C. and Bobak, I. M. 1977. *Maternity Care. The nurse and the family*. The C. V. Mosby Company, St Louis.

Jewson, N. 1993. Inequalities and Differences in Health. In Taylor, S. and Field, D. (eds), *Sociology of Health and Health Care: An introduction for nurses*. Ch. 4: pp. 57–93. Blackwell Scientific Publications Ltd, Oxford.

Johnston, R. L. 1989. Orem's Self Care Model for Nursing. In Fitzpatrick, J. J. and Whall, A. L. (eds), *Conceptual Models of Nursing*. 2nd Edition. Ch. 12: pp. 165–84. Appleton and Lange, Norwalk, Connecticut.

Josten, L. 1981. Prenatal Assessment Guide for Illuminating Possible Problems with Parenting. *MCN, The American Journal of Maternal Child Nursing* 6(2): 113–117

Jourard, S. M. 1971. *The Transparent Self*. 2nd Edition. D. Van Nostrand Company, New York.

Kane, R. 1990. The 'Line-Down-the-Middle' Theory of Nursing. *Nursing Forum* 25(3): 34–35.

Keane, J. 1982. The Nursing Process Applied to Midwifery. Volumes I and II. Diploma in Advanced Nursing Studies Dissertation. Unpublished. University of Manchester, Manchester.

Keck, J. F. 1989. Terminology of Theory Development. In Marriner-Tomey, A. (ed.), *Nursing Theorists and Their Work*. 2nd Edition. Ch. 2: pp. 15–23. The C. V. Mosby Company, St Louis.

Kershaw, B. and Salvage, J. (eds). 1986. *Models for Nursing*. John Wiley and Sons, Chichester.

Kesby, O. and Grant, M. 1985. Changing the System. *Nursing Mirror* 160(11): 28–31.

Khan, R. L., Wolfe, D. M., Quinn, R. P. and Snoek, J. D. 1964. *Organizational Stress: Studies in role conflict and ambiguity*. John Wiley and Sons, New York.

Kirkham, M. 1983. Labouring in the Dark: Limitations on the giving of information to enable patients to orientate themselves to the likely events and timescale of labour. In Wilson-Barnett, J. (ed.), *Nursing Research: Ten studies in patient care. Developments in nursing research*. Volume 2. Ch. 4: pp. 81–99. John Wiley and Sons, Chichester.

Kirkham, M. 1988. A Feminist Perspective in Midwifery. In Webb, C. (ed.), *Feminist Practice in Women's Health Care*. Ch. 3: pp. 35–49. John Wiley and Sons, Chichester.

Kirkham, M. 1989. Midwives and Information-giving during Labour. In Robinson, S. and Thomson, A. M. (eds), *Midwives, Research and Childbirth*. Vol I. Ch. 6: pp. 117–38. Chapman and Hall, London.

Kitson, A. 1993. *Nursing Art and Science*. Chapman and Hall, London.

Kitzinger, S. 1988. *The Midwife Challenge*. Pandora Press, London.

Kleinmann, A. 1980. *Patients and their Healers in the Context of Culture*. University of California Press, Berkeley. Cited by Littlewood, J. 1989. A Model for Nursing using Anthropological Literature. *International Journal of Nursing Studies* 26(3): 221–9.

Kloosterman, G. L. 1984. The Dutch Experience of Domiciliary Confinements. In Zander, L. and Chamberlain, G. (eds), *Pregnancy Care for the 1980s*. Ch. 13: pp. 115–25. Royal Society of Medicine and Macmillan, London.

Kolb, D. A. 1984. *Experiential Learning. Experience as the source of learning and development*. Prentice Hall, Englewood Cliffs, New Jersey.

Kuhn, T. 1962, 1970. *The Structure of Scientific Revolutions*. 2nd Edition. International Encyclopaedia of United Science, 2:2. The Chicago University

Press, Chicago. Cited in Robinson, J. 1992. Problems with paradigms in a caring profession. *Journal of Advanced Nursing* 17(5): 632–8.

Kwast, B. E. 1993. Safe Motherhood – the first decade. *Midwifery* 9(3): 105–23.

Lancaster, W. and Lancaster, J. 1992. Models and Model Building in Nursing. In Nicholl, L. H. (ed.) *Perspectives on Nursing Theory*. 2nd Edition. Ch. 42: pp. 432–41. J. B. Lippincott Company, Philadelphia.

Laryea, M. G. G. 1980. The Midwives' Role in the Postnatal Care of Primiparae and their Infants in the First 28 Days following Childbirth. MPhil thesis. Unpublished. Newcastle-upon-Tyne Polytechnic, Newcastle-upon-Tyne.

Leap, N. 1992. The Power of Words. *Nursing Times* 88(21): 60–1.

Leap, N. and Hunter, B. 1993. *The Midwife's Tale*. Scarlet Press, London.

Lehrman, E.-J. 1981. Nurse-Midwifery Practice: A Descriptive Study of Prenatal Care. *Journal of Nurse-Midwifery* 26(3): 27–41.

Lehrman, E.-J. 1988. A Theoretical Framework for Nurse-Midwifery Practice. PhD thesis. Unpublished. University of Arizona, Arizona.

Lehrman, E.-J. 1989. A Theoretical Framework for Nurse-Midwifery Practice. Dissertation Abstracts International 49(12): 5230-B.

Lehrman, E.-J. 1993. Personal communication.

Leong, W. C. 1989. The Introduction of Computer-assisted Learning in a School of Midwifery using the Wessex Care Plan Programme. *Nurse Education Today* 9(2): 114–23.

Levene, L. 1993. You Can't Go Wrong. *The Independent*, 9 August: 10.

Lewin, K. 1952. Group Decision and Social Change. In Swanson, G. E., Newcomb, T. M. and Hartley, E. L. (eds), *Readings in Social Psychology*. Revised Edition: pp. 459–73. Henry Holt and Company, New York.

Lewis, J. 1980. *The Politics of Motherhood: Child and Maternal Welfare in England, 1900–1939*. Croom Helm, London.

Littlewood, J. 1989. A Model for Nursing using Anthropological Literature. *International Journal of Nursing Studies* 26(3): 221–9.

Luker, K. 1988. Do Models Work? *Nursing Times* 84(5): 27–9.

Lynam, L. E. and Miller, M. A. 1991. Mothers' and Nurses' Perceptions of the Needs of Women Experiencing Preterm Labor. *JOGNN, Journal of Obstetric, Gynecologic and Neonatal Nursing* 21(2): 126–36.

MacArthur, C., Lewis, M. and Knox, E. G. 1991. *Health after Childbirth*. HMSO, London.

Macdonald, J. J. 1992. *Primary Health Care: Medicine in its place*. Earthscan, London.

MacFarlane, J. A. 1984. Facts, Beliefs and Misconceptions about the Bonding Process. In Zander, L. and Chamberlain, G. (eds), *Pregnancy Care for the 1980s*. Ch. 7: pp. 59–62. Royal Society of Medicine and Macmillan, London.

Macintyre, S. 1980. Interaction in Antenatal Clinics. In Robinson, S. (1981). (ed.), *'Research and the Midwife' Conference Proceedings* 1979 and 1980. Ch. 10: pp. 66–86. 'Research and the Midwife' Conference, London.

Maclean, G. 1993. 'Partnership in Care' – A tale of two African cities. *Modern Midwife* 3(3): 17–20.

Marriner-Tomey, A. (ed.) 1989. *Nursing Theorists and their Work*. 2nd Edition. The C. V. Mosby Company, St Louis.

Marris, P. 1986. *Loss and Change*. Routledge and Kegan Paul, London.

Martell, L. K. and Mitchell, S. K. 1984. Rubin's 'Puerperal Change' Reconsidered. *JOGNN, Journal of Obstetric, Gynecologic and Neonatal Nursing* 13(3): 145–9.

Marut, J. S. and Mercer, R. T. 1979. Comparison of Primiparas' Perceptions of Vaginal and Caesarean Births. *Nursing Research* 28(5): 260–6.

Maternity Services Advisory Committee. 1982. *Maternity Care in Action*. Part I: Antenatal Care. HMSO, London.

Maternity Services Advisory Committee, 1984. *Maternity Care in Action*. Part II: Care during Childbirth (Intrapartum Care). HMSO, London.

Maternity Services Advisory Committee. 1985. *Maternity Care in Action*. Part III: Care of the Mother and Baby (Postnatal Care). HMSO, London.

Mayes, G. E. 1987. Developing a model of midwifery care in Waltham Forest. *Midwives Chronicle* 100(1,198) Supplement: v–ix.

McBride, A. B. 1984. The Experience of Being a Parent. *Annual Review of Nursing Research* 2: 63–81. Cited by Bee, A. M. and Oetting, S. 1989. Ramona T Mercer: Maternal Role Attainment. In Marriner-Tomey, A. (ed.), *Nursing Theorists and Their Work*. 2nd Edition. Ch. 24: pp. 292–306. The C. V. Mosby Company, St Louis.

McCool, W. F. and McCool, S. J. 1989. Feminism and Nurse-Midwifery. Historical Overview and Current Issues. *Journal of Nurse-Midwifery* 34(6): 323–34.

McCrea, H. and Crute, V. 1991. Midwife/client Relationships: Midwives' perspectives. *Midwifery* 7(4): 183–92.

McCrea, H. 1993. Valuing the midwife's role in the midwife/client relationship. *Journal of Clinical Nursing* 2(1): 47–52.

McCrea, H. undated diary entry. Unpublished.

McDonald, M. 1986. Care Plan for a Woman in Labour and her Baby, based on Roper's Activities of Living model. In Webb, C. (ed.), *Women's Health: Midwifery and Gynaecological Nursing*. Ch. 4: pp. 70–96. Edward Arnold, London.

McKay, S. 1993. Models of Midwifery Care: Denmark, Sweden, and the Netherlands. *Journal of Nurse-Midwifery* 38(2): 114–20.

McKeown, T. 1989. *The Role of Medicine: Dream, Mirage or Nemesis?* Basil Blackwell, Oxford.

Mead, D. and Bryar, R. 1992. An analysis of the changes involved in the introduction of the nursing process and primary nursing using a theoretical framework of loss and attachment. *Journal of Clinical Nursing* 1(2): 95–9.

Menzies, I. E. P. 1970. *The Functioning of Social Systems as a Defence against Anxiety. A Report on the Nursing Service of a General Hospital*. Tavistock Institute of Human Relations, London.

Mercer, R. T. 1981a. The Nurse and Maternal Tasks of the Early Postpartum. *MCN, The American Journal of Maternal Child Nursing* 6(5): 341–5.

Mercer. R. T. 1981b. A Theoretical Framework for Studying the Factors that Impact on the Maternal Role. *Nursing Research* 30(2): 73–7.

Mercer, R. T. 1986. *First-Time Motherhood: Experiences from teens to forties.* Springer Publishing Company, New York.

Mercer, R. T., May, K. A., Ferketich, S. and DeJoseph, J. 1986. Theoretical Models for Studying the Effect of Antepartum Stress on the Family. *Nursing Research* 35(6): 339–46.

Mercer, R. T., Ferketich, S. L., DeJoseph, J., May, K. A. and Sollid, D. 1988. Effect of Stress on Family Functioning During Pregnancy. *Nursing Research* 37(5): 268–75.

Methven, R. 1982. An Examination of the Content and Process of the Antenatal Booking Interview (Recording an Obstetric History or Relating with a Mother-to-be?). MSc thesis. Unpublished. University of Manchester, Manchester.

Methven, R. C. 1986a. Care Plan for a Woman having Ante-natal Care, based on Orem's Self-care Model. In Webb, C. (ed.), *Women's Health: Midwifery and Gynaecological Nursing.* Ch. 2: pp. 13–41. Edward Arnold, London.

Methven, R. C. 1986b. Care Plan for a Woman during Pregnancy, Labour and the Puerperium, based on Henderson's Activities of Daily Living Model. In Webb, C. (ed.), *Women's Health. Midwifery and Gynaecological Nursing.* Ch. 3: pp. 42–69. Edward Arnold, London.

Methven, R. C. 1989. Recording an Obstetric History or Relating to a Pregnant Woman? A study of the antenatal booking interview. In Robinson, S. and Thomson, A. M. (eds), *Midwives, Research and Childbirth.* Volume I. Ch. 3: pp. 42–71. Chapman and Hall, London.

Methven, R. C. 1990. The Antenatal Booking Interview. In Alexander, J., Levy, V. and Roch, S. (eds), *Antenatal Care. A research-based approach.* Ch. 3: pp. 42–57. Macmillan, London.

Ministry of Welfare, Health and Cultural Affairs. 1987. *Health as a Focal Point.* An abridged version of the *Memorandum Health 2000: The Netherlands.* Ministry of Welfare, Health and Cultural Affairs, The Hague, The Netherlands.

Minshull, J., Ross, K. and Turner, J. 1986. The Human Needs Model of Nursing. *Journal of Advanced Nursing* 11(6): 643–9.

Moody, L. E. 1990. *Advancing Nursing Science through Research.* Volume I. SAGE Publications, Newbury Park.

Moore, M. L. 1983. *Realities in Childbearing.* 2nd Edition. W. B. Saunders Company, Philadelphia.

Morley, D., Rohde, J. and Williams, G. 1989. *Practising Health for All.* Oxford University Press, Oxford.

Morse, J. M. 1992. Editorial: If You Believe in Theories.... *Qualitative Health Research* 2(3): 259–61.

Morton, A., Kohl, M., O'Mahoney, P. and Pelosi, K. 1991. Certified Nurse-Midwifery Care of the Postpartum Client. *Journal of Nurse-Midwifery* 36(5): 276–88.

Morton-Cooper, A. and Palmer, A. 1993. *Mentoring and Preceptorship. A guide to support roles in clinical practice*. Blackwell Scientific Publications, Oxford.

Murphy-Black, T. and Faulkner, A. (eds). 1988. *Antenatal Group Skills Training. A Manual of Guidelines*. John Wiley and Sons, Chichester.

Murphy-Black, T. 1992a. *A Survey of Systems of Midwifery Care in Scotland*. Nursing Research Unit, Department of Nursing Studies, University of Edinburgh, Edinburgh.

Murphy-Black, T. 1992b. Systems of Midwifery Care in Use in Scotland. *Midwifery* 8(3): 113–24.

Myles, M. 1985. *Textbook for Midwives*. 10th Edition. Churchill Livingstone, Edinburgh.

National Childbirth Trust. 1981. *Change in Antenatal Care*. The National Childbirth Trust, London.

National Childbirth Trust. 1993. Winterton Action Pack. The National Childbirth Trust, London.

NHS Management Executive. 1992. *The Health of the Nation. First Steps for the NHS*. Department of Health, London.

NHS Management Executive. 1993. *A Study of Midwife-led and GP-led Maternity Units*. Department of Health, London.

Neuman, B. 1989. *The Neuman Systems Model*. 2nd Edition. Appleton and Lange, Norwalk, Connecticut.

New Zealand College of Midwives (Inc). 1992. *Midwives' Handbook for Practice*. New Zealand College of Midwives, Auckland.

Newburn, M. 1993. Choice, Continuity and Care. *New Generation*. June: 20–1.

Nickel, S., Gesse, T. and MacLaren, A. 1992. Ernestine Wiedenbach: Her professional legacy. *Journal of Nurse-Midwifery* 37(3): 161–7.

Nicoll, L. H. (ed.). 1992. *Perspectives on Nursing Theory*. 2nd Edition. J. B. Lippincott Company, Philadelphia.

Oakley, A. 1979. *Becoming a Mother*. Martin Robertson, Oxford.

Oakley, A. 1980. *Women Confined: Towards a sociology of childbirth*. Martin Robertson, Oxford.

Oakley, A. and Chamberlain, G. 1981. Medical and Social Factors in Postpartum Depression. *Journal of Obstetrics and Gynaecology* 1(3): 182–7.

Oakley, A., Rajan, L. and Grant, A. 1990. Social Support and Pregnancy Outcome. *British Journal of Obstetrics and Gynaecology* 97: 155–62.

Oakley, P. 1989. *Community Involvement in Health Development. An examination of the critical issues*. WHO, Geneva.

Odent, M. 1984. *Entering the World. The De-medicalisation of Childbirth*. Marion Boyars, London.

Offerman, J. 1985. The Netherlands. *Childbirth Education*, Fall: 26–31. Cited by Kitzinger, S. (ed.), *The Midwife Challenge*. Pandora, London.

O'Meara, C. M. 1993. A Diagnostic Model for the Evaluation of Childbirth and Parenting Education. *Midwifery* 9(1): 28–34.

Opoku, D. K. 1992. Does Inter-professional Co-operation Matter in the Care of the Birthing Woman? *Journal of Interprofessional Care* 6 (2): 119–25.

Oppenheimer, C. 1993. Organising Midwifery-led Care in the Netherlands. *British Medical Journal* 3,307: 1,400–2.

Owen, G. 1983. The Stress of Change. *Nursing Times* 79(4): 44–6.

Page, L. 1993. Redefining the Midwife's Role: Changes needed in practice. *British Journal of Midwifery* 1(1): 21–4.

Pallot, P. 1993. Home-birth Doctor Says Sack Half the Obstetricians. *Daily Telegraph* 13 October: 4.

Pearson, A. and Vaughan, B. 1986. *Nursing Models for Practice*. Heinemann Nursing, London.

Pearson, A. 1992. Knowing Nursing: Emerging paradigms in nursing. In Robinson, K. and Vaughan, B. 1992. *Knowledge for Nursing Practice*. Ch. 14: 213–26. Butterworth/Heinemann, Oxford.

Powell, J. H. 1989. The Reflective Practitioner in Nursing. *Journal of Advanced Nursing*. 14(10): 824–32.

Price, A. and Price, B. 1993. Midwifery Knowledge: Theory for action, theory for practice. *British Journal of Midwifery* 1(5): 233–7.

Pridham, K. F. and Chang, A. S. 1992. Transition to Being the Mother of a New Infant in the First 3 Months: Maternal problem solving and self-appraisals. *Journal of Advanced Nursing* 17(2): 204–16.

Prince, J. and Adams, M. E. 1987. *The Psychology of Childbirth: An introduction for mothers and midwives*. 2nd Edition. Churchill Livingstone, Edinburgh.

Quillan, J. A. and Runk, S. I. M. 1989. Martha Rogers' Unitary Person Model. In Fitzpatrick, J. J. and Whall, A. L. (eds), *Conceptual Models of Nursing*. 2nd Edition. Ch. 19: pp. 285–300. Appleton and Lange, Norwalk, Connecticut.

Rambo, B. J. 1984. *Adaptation Nursing Assessment and Intervention*. W. B. Saunders Company, Philadelphia.

Raleigh, E. D. 1989. Wiedenbach's Model of Nursing Practice. In Fitzpatrick, J. J. and Whall, A. L. (eds), *Conceptual Models of Nursing*. Ch. 7: pp. 89–107. Appleton and Lange, Norwalk, Connecticut.

Rees van S., Smulders, B., Limburg, A. and Kloosterman, G. J. 1984. *Giving Birth*. Stichting Lichaamstaal, Leveroy, The Netherlands.

Rhoades, J. M. 1989. Social Support and the Transition to the Maternal Role. In Stern, P. S. (ed.), *Pregnancy and Parenting*. Ch. 10: pp. 131–41. Hemisphere Publishing Corporation, New York.

Rhodes, J. M. R. 1988. Integrating Philosophy into the Doctoral Preparation for Nurse-Midwives. *Journal of Nurse-Midwifery* 33(6): 283–4.

Richards, M. 1984. The Myth of Bonding. In Zander, L. and Chamberlain, G. (eds), *Pregnancy Care for the 1980s*. Ch. 6: pp. 51–8. Royal Society of Medicine and Macmillan, London.

Rifkin, S. B. 1990. *Community Participation in Maternal and Child Health/Family Planning Programmes*. WHO, Geneva.

Roach, M. and Brown, N. 1991. Using Riehl's Model in Midwifery. *Nursing Standard* 5(32): 24–6.

Roberts, E. 1984. *A Woman's Place. An Oral History of Working-Class Women, 1890–1940*. Basil Blackwell, Oxford.

Robinson, J. A. 1992. Problems with Paradigms in a Caring Profession. *Journal of Advanced Nursing* 17(5): 632–8.

Robinson, K. and Vaughan, B. 1992. *Knowledge for Nursing Practice.* Butterworth/Heinemann, Oxford.

Robinson, S., Golden, J. and Bradley, S. 1983. *A Study of the Role and Responsibilities of the Midwife.* Nursing Education Research Unit Report Number 1. Nursing Education Research Unit, King's College, London.

Robinson, S. 1985. Midwives, Obstetricians and General Practitioners: The need for role clarification. *Midwifery* 1(2): 102–13.

Rogers, C. R. 1961. *On Becoming a Person: A therapist's view of psychotherapy.* Houghton Mifflin, Boston. Cited in Morton, A., Kohl, M., O'Mahoney, P. and Pelosi, K. 1991. Certified Nurse-Midwifery Care of the Postpartum Client. *Journal of Nurse-Midwifery* 36(5): 276–88.

Romney, M. and White, V. J. L. 1984. Current Practices in Labour. In Field, P. A. (ed.), Recent Advances in Nursing 8. *Perinatal Nursing.* Ch. 4: pp. 63–80. Churchill Livingstone, Edinburgh.

Roper, N., Logan, W. W. and Tierney, A. J. 1981. *Learning to Use the Process of Nursing.* Churchill Livingstone, Edinburgh.

Roper, N., Logan, W. W. and Tierney, A. J. 1983. (eds), *Using a Model for Nursing.* Churchill Livingstone, Edinburgh.

Roper, N., Logan, W. W. and Tierney, A. J. 1985. *The Elements of Nursing.* 2nd Edition. Churchill Livingstone, Edinburgh.

Rothman, B. K. 1983. Midwives in Transition: The Structure of a Clinical Revolution. *Social Problems* 30(3): pp. 262–71.

Royal College of Midwives. 1991. Towards a Healthy Nation: Every day a birth day. Royal College of Midwives, London.

Royal College of Nursing. 1993. *Standards of Care for Midwifery.* RCN Standards of Care Project. RCN, London.

Royal College of Obstetricians and Gynaecologists. 1982. *Report of the RCOG Working Party on Antenatal and Intrapartum Care.* RCOG, London. Cited by Opoku, D. 1992. Does Interprofessional Co-operation Matter in the Care of Birthing Women? *Journal of Interprofessional Care.* 6(2): 119–25.

Rubin, R. 1961. Puerperal Change. *Nursing Outlook* 9(12): 743–55.

Rubin, R. 1967a. Attainment of the Maternal Role. Part I. Processes. *Nursing Research* 16(3): 237–45.

Rubin, R. 1967b. Attainment of the Maternal Role. Part II. Models and Referrants. *Nursing Research* 16(4): 342–6.

Rubin, R. 1984. Maternal Identity and the Maternal Experience. Springer Publishing Co, Inc., New York.

Russell, B. 1930. Cited by Khan, R. L., Wolfe, D. M., Quinn, R. P. and Snoek, J. D. 1964. *Organizational Stress: Studies in role conflict and ambiguity.* John Wiley and Sons, New York.

Salariya, E. 1990. Parental–infant attachment. In Alexander, J., Levy, V. and Roch, S. (eds), *Postnatal Care. A research-based approach.* Ch. 4: pp. 62–83. Macmillan, London.

Salford Community Health Council. 1992. How Far Does Choice Extend? Choices in Maternity Care for Women in Salford. *Association of Radical Midwives Midwifery Matters* 55(Winter): 8–9.

Schein, E. H. 1972. *Professional Education: Some new directions.* McGraw-Hill, New York.

Schön, D. A. 1983. *The Reflective Practitioner: How professionals think in action.* Basic Books, HarperCollins, London.

Schön, D. A. 1992. The Crisis of Professional Knowledge and the Pursuit of an Epistemology of Practice. *Journal of Interprofessional Care* 6 (1): 49–63.

Shorney, J. 1990. Preconception Care – the embryo of health promotion. In Alexander, J., Levy, V. and Roch, S. (eds), *Antenatal Care. A research-based approach.* Ch. 1: pp. 1–19. Macmillan, London.

Sills, D. L. (ed.), 1972. *International Encyclopaedia of the Social Sciences.* Volumes 3 and 4. The Macmillan Co. and The Free Press, New York.

Silva, M. 1981. Selection of a Theoretical Framework. In Krampitz, S. D. and Pavlovich, N. (eds), Readings for Nursing Research. C. V. Mosby, St Louis. Cited in Moody, L. E. 1990. *Advancing Nursing Science Through Research.* Volume 1. SAGE Publications, Newbury Park.

Silverman, D. 1970. *The Theory of Organisations.* Heinemann, London.

Silverton, L. 1993. *The Art and Science of Midwifery.* Prentice Hall, New York.

Simpson, J. A. and Weiner, E. S. C. (eds). 1989. *The Oxford English Dictionary.* 2nd Edition. Clarendon Press, Oxford.

Smith, A. and Jacobson, B. 1988. *The Nation's Health: A Strategy for the 1990s.* King Edward's Hospital Fund for London, London.

Smith, A. 1991. Newbourne Optimism. *Nursing Times* 87(16): 56–9.

Smith, P. 1992. *The Emotional Labour of Nursing.* Macmillan, London.

Smulders, B. and Limburg, A. 1988. Obstetrics and Midwifery in the Netherlands. In Kitzinger, S. (ed.), *The Midwife Challenge.* Ch. 12: pp. 235–49. Pandora Press, London.

Spires, L. 1991. A Model for Midwifery Practice? *Modern Midwife* 1(5): 9–11.

Stacey, M. 1988. *The Sociology of Health and Healing. A Textbook.* Routledge, London.

Strauss, A., Schatzman, L., Bucher, R., Ehrlich, D. and Sabshin, A. 1964. *Psychiatric Ideologies and Institutions.* The Free Press of Glencoe, Collier-Macmillan, London.

Sullivan, D. A. and Weitz, R. 1988. *Labor Pains. Modern midwives and home birth.* Yale University Press, New Haven.

Taylor, B. J. 1992. From Helper to Human: A reconceptualization of the nurse as a person. *Journal of Advanced Nursing* 17(9): 1042–9.

Taylor, E. M. and Coventry, M. 1983. A Midwife's Study of a Mother and Baby using the Model for Nursing. In Roper, N., Logan, W. W. and Tierney, A. J. (eds), *Using a Model for Nursing.* Ch. 6: pp. 68–78. Churchill Livingstone, Edinburgh.

Teijlingen, van E. R. and McCaffery, P. 1987. The Profession of Midwife in the Netherlands. *Midwifery* 3(4): 178–86.

Teijlingen, van E. R. 1990. The Profession of Maternity Home Care Assistant and Its Significance for the Dutch Midwifery Profession. *International Journal of Nursing Studies* 27(4): 355–66.

Teijlingen, van E. R. 1991. Comparing the Dutch and British Organisation of Maternity Care: Long-term Consequences of State Intervention. Unpublished paper, International Conference of Primary Care Obstetrics and Perinatal Health: Quality Assessment in Different Settings, s'Hertogenbosch, The Netherlands, March.

Teijlingen, van E. R. 1992. The Organisation of Maternity Care in the Netherlands. *The Association for Community-based Maternity Care Newsletter* No. 5: 2–4.

Teijlingen, van E. R. 1993. Personal communication.

Telfer, F. M. 1990. Identification and Analysis of the Health Education Needs of Young Pregnant Women. MSc dissertation. Unpublished. University of Manchester, Manchester.

Telfer, F. M. 1991. A Framework for Midwifery Care Contingent on Need. Unpublished, Mid Trent College of Nursing and Midwifery, Faculty of Midwifery.

Telfer, F. M. 1993. Personal communication.

Thompson, J. E., Oakley, D., Burke, M., Jay, S. and Conklin, M. 1989. Theory Building in Nurse-Midwifery. The Care Process. *Journal of Nurse-Midwifery* 34(3): 120–30.

Thomson, A. M. 1980. Planned or Unplanned? Are Midwives Ready for the 1980s? *Midwives Chronicle and Nursing Notes* 93(1,106): 68–72.

Tiedeman, M. E. 1989. The Roy Adaptation Model. In Fitzpatrick, J. J. and Whall, A. L. (eds), *Conceptual Models for Nursing*. 2nd Edition. Ch. 13: pp. 185–204. Appleton and Lange, Norwalk, Connecticut.

Tiran, D. and Nunnerley. R. 1986. Untangling the Midwifery Process with COMB – Care of Mothers and Babies. *Midwives Chronicle* 99(1,184): 208–11.

Titcombe, H. 1991. Empowering Women. In South East Thames Regional Health Authority, *Power to the People in South East Thames*. A Conference about Empowering the Patient 11 November 1991: 49–51. South East Thames Regional Health Authority, Bexhill-on-Sea.

Towler, J. and Butler-Manuel, R. 1980. *Modern Obstetrics for Student Midwives*. 2nd Edition, Lloyd-Luke (Medical Books), London.

Towler, J. and Bramall, J. 1986. *Midwives in History and Society*. Croom Helm, London.

UNICEF 1990a. *Facts for Life. Communication Challenge*. UNICEF, New York.

UNICEF 1990b. *All for Health. A resource book for Facts for Life*. UNICEF, New York.

Vaughan, B. 1992. The Nature of Nursing Knowledge. In Robinson, R. and Vaughan, B. 1992. *Knowledge for Nursing Practice*. Ch. 1: pp. 3–19. Butterworth/Heinemann, London.

Vouri, H. and Rimpela, M. 1981. The Development and Impact of the Medical Model. *Perspectives in Biology and Medicine*. Winter: 217–28.

Walker, J. F. 1976. Midwife or Obstetric Nurse? Some perceptions of mid-wives and obstetricians of the role of the midwife. *Journal of Advanced Nursing* 1(2): 129–38.

Walker, R. 1991. Midwifery. The dream and the reality. *Midwives Chronicle and Nursing Notes* 104(1,246): 330–2.

Warrier, S. 1991. Finding out About Consumer Perceptions. In South East Thames Regional Health Authority, *Power to the People in South East Thames*. A Conference about Empowering the Patient, 11 November 1991: 34–6. South East Thames Regional Health Authority, Bexhill-on-Sea.

Waterhouse, I. 1989. Oh to be a Midwife: The Reading model. *Midwife, Health Visitor and Community Nurse* 25(9): 395–6.

Webb, C. (ed.). 1986. *Women's Health. Midwifery and gynaecological nursing*. Edward Arnold, London.

Weber, M. 1957. *The Theory of Social and Economic Organizations*. Collier-Macmillan, London.

Weitz, R. and Sullivan, D. 1985. Licensed Lay Midwifery and the Medical Model of Childbirth. *Sociology of Health and Illness* 7(1): 36–54.

Welford, H. 1993. A Room of One's Own. *Modern Midwife* 3(5): 34–5.

Welsh Health Planning Forum. 1991. *Protocol for Investment in Health Gain: Maternal and early child health*. Welsh Office, Cardiff.

Wessel, H. and Ellis, H. F. (eds). 1987. Childbirth without Fear: The original approach to natural childbirth, Grantley Dick-Read. 5th Edition. Harper and Row, New York.

West Glamorgan Health Authority. 1992. Standards of Midwifery Practice. West Glamorgan Health Authority, Swansea.

Whall, A. L. 1989. Nursing Theory Issues and Debates. In Fitzpatrick, J. J. and Whall, A. L. (eds), *Conceptual Models of Nursing. Analysis and Application*. 2nd Edition. Ch. 2: pp. 15–22. Appleton and Lange, Norwalk, Connecticut.

Whitfield, S. 1983. Sir William Powell Memorial Lecture: The midwifery process in practice. *Midwives Chronicle* 96(1145): 186–9.

Wiedenbach, E. 1949. Childbirth as Mothers Say They Like It. *Public Health Nursing* 5: 417–21.

Wiedenbach, E. 1960. Nurse-Midwifery: Purpose, Practice and Opportunity. *Nursing Outlook* 8(5): 256–9.

Wiedenbach, E. 1964. Clinical Nursing: A helping art. Springer, New York.

Wiedenbach, E. 1967. Family-Centred Maternity Nursing. G. P. Putnam's Sons, New York.

World Health Organization. 1981. *Global Strategy for Health for All by the Year 2000*. WHO, Geneva.

World Health Organization. 1985a. *Having a Baby in Europe*. Public Health in Europe 26. WHO, Copenhagen.

World Health Organization. 1985b. *Targets for Health for All. Targets in support of the European regional strategy for health for all*. WHO, Copenhagen.

World Health Organization. 1988. *From Alma-Ata to the Year 2000. Reflections at the midpoint*. WHO, Geneva.

World Health Organization. 1989. *Nursing in Primary Health Care: Ten Years after Alma-Ata and Perspectives for the Future*. Report of the Joint WHO/ICN Consultation. WHO, Geneva.

World Health Organization. 1990. *Human Resource Development for Maternal Health and Safe Motherhood*. WHO, Geneva.

World Health Organization. 1991. *Community Involvement in Health Development: Challenging health services: Report of a WHO study group*. WHO Technical Report Series No. 809. WHO, Geneva.

World Health Organization. 1992. *Training of Traditional Birth Attendants (TBAs). A guide for TBA trainers*. WHO, Geneva.

Wraight, A., Ball, J., Seccombe, I. and Stock, J. 1993. *Mapping Team Midwifery*. IMS Report Series 242. Institute of Manpower Studies, University of Sussex, Brighton.

Wright, S. 1986. Developing and Using a Nursing Model. In Kershaw, B. and Salvage, J. (eds), *Models for Nursing*. Ch. 5: pp. 39–46. John Wiley and Sons, Chichester.

Wright, S. 1990. *Building and Using a Model for Nursing*. 2nd Edition. Edward Arnold, London.

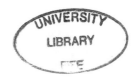